Fibromyalgia: Your Treatment Guide

Christine Craggs-Hinton, mother of three, followed a career in the Civil Service until, in 1991, she developed fibromyalgia, a chronic pain condition. Christine took up writing for therapeutic reasons and has, in the past few years, produced more than a dozen health-related self-help books for Sheldon Press. She also writes for the Fibromyalgia Association UK and the UK Fibromyalgia magazine called *FaMily*. A few years ago, Christine and her husband moved to the Canary Islands where she works as the agony aunt and health writer for a local newspaper.

D0417262

Overcoming Common Problems Series

Selected titles

A full list of titles is available from Sheldon Press,
36 Causton Street, London SW1P 4ST and on our website at
www.sheldonpress.co.uk

101 Questions to Ask Your Doctor
Dr Tom Smith

Birth Over 35
Sheila Kitzinger

Coeliac Disease: What you need to know
Alex Gazzola

**Coping Successfully with Chronic Illness:
Your healing pain**
Neville Shone

Coping Successfully with Shyness
Margaret Oakes, Professor Robert Bor
and Dr Carina Eriksen

Coping with Anaemia
Dr Tom Smith

Coping with Asthma in Adults
Mark Greener

Coping wth Bronchitis and Emphysema
Dr Tom Smith

Coping with Drug Problems in the Family
Lucy Jolin

Coping with Early-onset Dementia
Jill Eckersley

Coping with Eating Disorders and Body Image
Christine Craggs-Hinton

Coping with Gout
Christine Craggs-Hinton

**Coping with Manipulation: When others
blame you for their feelings**
Dr Windy Dryden

**Coping with Obsessive Compulsive
Disorder**
Professor Kevin Gournay, Rachel Piper
and Professor Paul Rogers

Coping with Stomach Ulcers
Dr Tom Smith

Depressive Illness: The curse of the strong
Dr Tim Cantopher

The Diabetes Healing Diet
Mark Greener and Christine Craggs-Hinton

Dying for a Drink
Dr Tim Cantopher

**Epilepsy: Complementary and alternative
treatments**
Dr Sallie Baxendale

Fibromyalgia: Your Treatment Guide
Christine Craggs-Hinton

The Heart Attack Survival Guide
Mark Greener

How to Beat Worry and Stress
Dr David Devlin

How to Come Out of Your Comfort Zone
Dr Windy Dryden

How to Develop Inner Strength
Dr Windy Dryden

How to Eat Well When You Have Cancer
Jane Freeman

**Let's Stay Together: A guide to lasting
relationships**
Jane Butterworth

Living with IBS
Nuno Ferreira and David T. Gillanders

Losing a Parent
Fiona Marshall

Making Sense of Trauma: How to tell your story
Dr Nigel C. Hunt and Dr Sue McHale

Motor Neurone Disease: A family affair
Dr David Oliver

Natural Treatment for Arthritis
Christine Craggs-Hinton

Overcoming Loneliness
Alice Muir

**The Pain Management Handbook:
Your personal guide**
Neville Shone

The Panic Workbook
Dr Carina Eriksen, Professor Robert Bor
and Margaret Oakes

Reducing Your Risk of Dementia
Dr Tom Smith

**Therapy for Beginners: How to get the best
out of counselling**
Professor Robert Bor, Sheila Gill and Anne Stokes

**Transforming Eight Deadly Emotions
into Healthy Ones**
Dr Windy Dryden

Treating Arthritis: The drug-free way
Margaret Hills and Christine Horner

Treating Arthritis: The supplements guide
Julia Davies

**When Someone You Love Has Depression:
A handbook for family and friends**
Barbara Baker

Overcoming Common Problems

Fibromyalgia:
Your Treatment Guide

CHRISTINE CRAGGS-HINTON

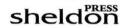

First published in Great Britain in 2013

Sheldon Press
36 Causton Street
London SW1P 4ST
www.sheldonpress.co.uk

British Library Cataloguing-in-Publication Data
A catalogue record for this book is available from the British Library

ISBN 978–1–84709–244–1
eBook ISBN 978–1–84709–245–8

Typeset by Caroline Waldron, Wirral, Cheshire
First printed in Great Britain by Ashford Colour Press
Subsequently digitally printed in Great Britain

Produced on paper from sustainable forests

Contents

I thank you all for the wonderful feedback I received from my previous fibromyalgia books – it has inspired me to write this one. I know from personal experience how challenging life is when you have fibromyalgia, and I have worked hard to give my very best help and advice. Don't ever think you have tried every option. There is always another door to open, somewhere along the way.

Note to the reader

Every effort has been made to ensure that the information in this book is accurate and current at the time of publication. The author and the publisher cannot accept responsibility for any misuse or misunderstanding of any information contained herein. The opinions and suggestions in this book are not intended to replace medical opinion. Indeed, the overview of prescription drugs is intended only to familiarize you with the medications most commonly prescribed for fibromyalgia and with those that are newly developed. This information is certainly not meant to replace medical advice and treatment. If you have concerns about your health, please seek a professional opinion.

We now suspect that the biblical Job had fibromyalgia. He wrote:

> I have been allotted months of futility, and nights of misery have been assigned to me. When I lie down I think, 'How long before I get up?' The night drags on, and I toss and turn until dawn . . . And now my life ebbs away; days of suffering grip me. Night pierces my bones; my gnawing pains never rest.
>
> (Job 7.3–4; 30.16–17)

Introduction

Good health is something we take for granted, until we no longer have it. A small percentage of us develop long-term conditions such as fibromyalgia in which we hurt all over, feel lacklustre and tired, find it difficult to achieve anything and can feel out of control. The best treatment strategy is not to fight the illness, but to go along with its demands until you have armed yourself with the tools with which to make positive changes. The best tool you can have available is self-education, where you learn for yourself as much as possible about what's wrong and find out what can be done for the very best outcome. Then inch by inch, step by step, you can move towards taking control once more.

Taking control involves learning how to use 'pacing' so you don't overtax yourself, thinking twice before committing yourself, and turning 'should do', 'ought to do' and 'must do' into 'will maybe do' or, better still, 'I'll see how things go before I make a decision'. For the people who ignore the challenge of making positive changes to their lives – lives that must, for now, incorporate a certain amount of pain – every action is a chore, every thought may be dark. Those people are also liable to move further away from getting back their lives.

Living with fibromyalgia isn't easy, as I myself know. It's a trial to change patterns of thinking and behaving, it's a trial to motivate ourselves to eat more healthily and start a gentle exercise routine. It doesn't help that when we make the effort to exercise we are rewarded by increased pain the next day and have no choice but to stay in bed, perhaps for weeks. Neither does it help that when we take the recommended medications and herbal remedies, we react badly and have to give them up. Is it worth all the effort, we might ask ourselves. We know deep down, though, that it is, for we are more than a bunch of symptoms, more than the façade we present to the world. We should therefore not only acknowledge the things that are important to us, but also think of things we *can* do, that are within our scope, that help us feel good about ourselves. Achievements, whether they are large or tiny, add positivity to life, raise our self-esteem and make us feel less of a drain on others.

I have had fibromyalgia for 20 years now, and in the early years struggled to accept the new me – that is, the me who could no longer work, 'play' or be relaxed with the people around me. The unremitting pain, which filled my mind as well as my body, was at last tempered by a series of analgesic trigger point injections, and in the pain lull I experienced I steeled myself to start using the pacing technique. This meant listening to my body, being careful not to overdo things and incorporating regular rest periods into my day. I also improved my diet and embarked upon an exercise routine, self-tailored to my particular strengths and weaknesses. And how well I remember the way my body suffered in response, the despondency I felt, the fear I succumbed to at the thought of trying to exercise again; but I succeeded in the end. I had to start out in a ridiculously small way – just circling my shoulders, then raising each arm in turn to the level of my head, making sure to rest afterwards. It took two or three years to significantly build up from there, and although my daily session still consists mainly of simple stretches, I spend 20 minutes doing them, which would have seemed miraculous before. Even more impressive is the fact that I can walk up to four miles once a week, which I usually do, with shorter walks in between.

Yes, exercise has made a great difference to my health and stamina, as has pacing and eating mainly a nutritious, well-balanced diet. Actually, lots of things in combination have helped, such as the medications I take, the positive outlook I've tried to adopt, as well as lots of smaller things – all of which combine to make my life more fulfilling. I doubt that I would have written 20 books if I hadn't had fibromyalgia, but once I began looking for something to attempt within my physical scope, writing seemed my obvious choice. You see, not only have I always loved writing, but I was taught to touch type at school, so I wouldn't need to strain my neck in looking down at the keyboard. I only hope that the things I have learned over the years can be of some benefit to others.

This book contains information about the neurological dysfunctions in fibromyalgia, and details of the best medications and self-help therapies currently available. It also discusses advances in the field and most promising treatments of tomorrow. The numerous symptoms associated with fibromyalgia are explored, with advice on how best to treat each one.

When one door closes, another opens; but we often look so long and so regretfully upon the closed door that we do not see the one which has opened for us.   (Alexander Graham Bell)

1

Fibromyalgia – an overview

Fibromyalgia syndrome is a chronic (long-term) pain disorder. It is characterized by the following:

- a lowered pain threshold
- diffuse pain in the muscles, tendons and ligaments (the soft tissues)
- extreme tenderness in certain areas
- difficulty achieving restorative sleep
- fatigue
- an array of sensitivity problems, such as dry mouth, dry eyes, food intolerances, chemical sensitivities, sensitivity to certain medications, sensitivity to cold or heat
- miscellaneous additional symptoms such as irritable bowel syndrome, irritable bladder, headaches, anxiety and depression.

The primary symptom of fibromyalgia is persistent pain in the soft fibrous tissues, namely the muscles, tendons and ligaments. Fortunately, the joints are not involved, and there is generally no soft tissue inflammation. The disorder is not degenerative either, which means that unlike most other pain conditions, you do not automatically get worse. Neither is there any evidence of it reducing lifespan. This doesn't mean that fibromyalgia (sometimes known as FM, for short) is not a serious condition – it can be, for the symptoms are incapacitating in a number of cases.

The pain of fibromyalgia can arise anywhere in the body. Some people say that at times they 'hurt all over', and at other times the bulk of the pain migrates from one area to another, for no obvious reason. However, it's slightly more common to have specific problem areas, which are usually those favoured in some way or temporarily subjected to a certain amount of stress. As a consequence, the muscles feel as if they have been 'pulled' or overworked. The shoulder and arm of a person with fibromyalgia may throb and burn, for instance, after carrying home a bag of shopping or simply reaching up to take a jar from a shelf. Some people with fibromyalgia experience extreme soreness after carrying out the smallest of tasks, the slightest of movements, which clearly has significant impact on their emotional state and quality of life. Others, though, if they employ great care, are able to hold down a paying job and enjoy a fairly good social life.

The word fibromyalgia is made up from 'fibro', meaning fibrous tissues such as the tendons and ligaments, 'my' meaning muscles, and 'algia' meaning pain. The term fibromyalgia has been used for over 30 years; before that the condition was known as fibrositis or rheumatism. It must be said, though, that 'fibromyalgia' doesn't accurately describe the condition, for although the pain is felt in the soft tissues in the peripheral (outer) areas of the body, there is no evidence that it arises as a result of problems there. Researchers actually believe that the symptoms come from subtle changes in hormones in the brain and central nervous system. I will discuss these hormones in more detail in further chapters.

Just as each person the world over is different, fibromyalgia is experienced differently by each individual, no matter where they come from or what they do. However, one thing we all have in common is that our pain is an exaggerated response to whatever stimulus caused it, an overreaction in protest to carrying out work. The condition reminds me of a hormonal adolescent throwing a tantrum after being made to do a job! Adolescents grow out of this phase as their hormones settle down, but there's no such luck with fibromyalgia. Our hormones remain out of balance and continue giving the overreaction. Indeed, fibromyalgia is, in most cases, a fixed, persisting condition for which there is as yet no absolute cure. It's only fortunate that there are many treatments of both the chemical and natural variety that can vastly reduce the condition's severity, and these are the focus of this book.

The full name of our condition is 'fibromyalgia syndrome' – the word 'syndrome' meaning that the disorder comprises several health problems, all neatly wrapped up with the one label slapped on it (see pages 49–74 for information about symptoms). Pain is obviously the main symptom – the one posing the greatest challenge – but there are many more associated health issues, which vary considerably from person to person and come and go over time. Given the right treatment, some symptoms disappear altogether in many people.

A sudden exacerbation of symptoms is known as a flare-up. Medical professionals say that on average most people have two major flare-ups a year, lasting around one month each time. However, some of us have repeated flare-ups while others go a full year without one. The situations most likely to trigger a flare-up are probably known to you quite well already. They are:

- when your stress levels are high;
- when you have overexerted yourself;
- in changes of weather, usually when the temperature drops or it becomes quite damp – for some people, a change to hot, muggy weather is a trigger.

Because symptoms can be numerous, and on the face of it unrelated, it's not unusual for people with fibromyalgia to suspect others believe they are hypochondriacs. It doesn't help that no one, not even close friends and family, can actually see how much we hurt, the exhaustion, the headaches, the brain fog, the dry eyes and mouth. And because fibromyalgia is an invisible condition, other people may struggle to trust our explanations. They can even suspect that we're 'putting some of it on', or even 'faking it' altogether, perhaps for attention. If, like me, you have encountered suspicion, you'll know how distressing it is. But when the people around begin to understand, to take you at your word, the relief is terrific. It's even greater when the medical profession finally presents you with a name for your 'problems', for it feels that at last there's a real and solid reason for the way you feel. Now you can actually tell people what's wrong, ask them to read about the condition on the internet, or even loan them a book on the subject.

The typical delay in diagnosis is often due to the tremendous variability in fibromyalgia symptoms between one patient and another. The symptoms can, in fact, give rise to a great deal of medical perplexity. We can only be thankful that, in the main, our medical professionals now know much more about the condition and are increasingly aware of how common it is. As a result, correct diagnoses are being arrived at much earlier than ever before.

Statistics from rheumatology clinics indicate that the prevalence of fibromyalgia ranges from 1.3 to 7.3 per cent of the population. Statistics also show that the condition is seven times more likely to occur in women than in men, which is probably owing to hormonal differences between the sexes.

Happily, fibromyalgia is one of the few long-term conditions where very positive results can be seen. These results have to be worked for, however. People who do nothing to improve their condition may only get worse over time. Medical help is no doubt of great importance, but whether we improve or not can depend on our own attitudes and behaviour. I understand very well that some unexpected sledgehammer can knock us down at any time – that's fibromyalgia. It's how we respond to such an 'attack' that seems to matter, in the majority of cases.

Fibromyalgia symptoms

The chief symptoms linked with fibromyalgia include the following:

- persistent soft tissue pain
- sleep problems and fatigue
- anxiety and depression
- irritable bowel syndrome and irritable bladder
- headaches and migraine
- multiple sensitivities in relation to chemicals, food, medications
- foggy brain (causing memory loss, poor concentration, word mix-ups and so on).

See Chapter 2 for in-depth information about fibromyalgia symptoms.

Why does fibromyalgia arise?

As fibromyalgia often occurs following physically or emotionally stressful events, it has been described as a 'stress syndrome'. The condition is certainly exacerbated by such things. In my own case, a whiplash injury incurred in a traffic accident triggered repeated problems in my neck, such as trapped nerves, and on two occasions a prolapsed vertebral disc. At the same time I was incredibly stressed due to a failing marriage. I therefore experienced both physical and emotional stressors prior to fibromyalgia taking hold. I suspect that the greater the stressors, the more severe is the resultant fibromyalgia.

The main triggers of fibromyalgia are now thought to be as follows:

- *Genetics* – according to various studies, fibromyalgia is common in families, often following the female line and sometimes skipping a generation. Researchers have concluded that if one parent has fibromyalgia, the female offspring have a 50 per cent chance of developing it, but only if they experience a triggering incident. Important research into the influence of genes and environment on the development of fibromyalgia is now under way and we hope to have the results quite soon.

- *Trauma* – an injury is often the triggering factor, and a whiplash injury is 13 times more likely to result in fibromyalgia than an injury in other areas. The trauma is believed to instigate neuro-logical and biochemical changes in first the muscle and then the central nervous system (which consists of the spinal cord and brain). The outcome is chronic pain, as described in greater detail in later pages. Fibromyalgia caused by trauma is known as post-traumatic fibromyalgia.
- *Extreme stress* – when an individual is subjected to extreme stress for a prolonged period, the hormones get out of balance and start to amplify pain.
- *Rheumatic and connective tissue disorders* – 'secondary' fibro-myalgia can arise when certain disorders are already present. Such disorders include rheumatoid arthritis, polymyalgia rheumatica, Sjögren's syndrome and lupus. The reason why secondary fibromyalgia arises may be genetic in nature. Some experts link its development to chemical exposure.
- *Infection* – in some cases, fibromyalgia is apparently triggered by a viral infection such as influenza, bronchitis, the Epstein-Barr virus and even the common cold. Yeast infections, parasite infections, the human Herpes 6 virus and salmonella can also be triggers. The subsequent inflammatory or autoimmune changes may start the nosedive into fibromyalgia.
- *Chemical exposure* – inhalation of certain toxic chemical fumes can be a trigger. Experts believe that the exposure causes the body to become overburdened, bringing about changes in the pain processing centres and upsetting hormone levels. The cul-prits are often vaccinations, pesticides, petroleum oils, paint thinner, cleaning solvents, dyes, gases and fumes, and agents used in chemical warfare.

Muscle spasm

If you have fibromyalgia and have experienced an injury, or managed to overwork one part of your body, the result is often a muscle spasm in that area, meaning a tight and painful contraction (squeezing) of the muscles. Muscle spasms are the body's means of protecting a damaged area, limiting movement until the area repairs itself. Unfortunately, in fibromyalgia the repair work can take place incredibly slowly, making the spasm reluctant to release its grip. Sometimes a bunch of muscles in spasm will trap a nearby nerve and 'refer' pain and perhaps numbness to a further area – for example, a trapped nerve in your lower back can send a sharp pain down one leg and cause some numbness, and a trapped nerve in your shoulder can cause prickling and numbness in your fingers.

Unfortunately, prolonged muscle spasm causes the muscles to become ropy in consistency. They lose their natural elasticity and ability to become energized, making us feel very weak. When the muscles are then used in any way, they protest very strongly, sending out a burning, throbbing type of pain. Normal muscles, on the other hand, are soft, smooth and feel like strips of gelatine. They receive plenty of oxygen, glucose and other nutrients and quickly recover after use.

Many people with fibromyalgia are able to improve their condition by having regular massages, hot and cold therapy, carrying out an exercise routine and so on. They often find that the spasm returns surprisingly easily, though, on overworking the muscles. It takes a dedicated regime of pacing, exercise and various other treatments to gradually strengthen the muscles so that they no longer respond so disastrously to overwork. The advice in this book is largely aimed at strengthening your muscles so that they are more able to cope with the demands of a reasonably normal lifestyle.

Diagnosing fibromyalgia

As yet, no laboratory tests are capable of diagnosing fibromyalgia. Your doctor has no choice but to listen to you, observe you, examine you and use his or her medical knowledge, fitting together the pieces jigsaw-style – hopefully correctly – to make a clear picture.

To help your doctor assemble the right picture, he or she needs to know all your symptoms. You must therefore make sure that you relate exactly how you have been feeling in the last three months; write down things beforehand if that will help. Your problems may appear vastly unrelated to you, but to your doctor with his or her medical training and ongoing medical reading (one hopes), the pieces should gradually slot together, precisely as they should.

In the physical examination, your tender points will be assessed. Swellings, spasm and weakness will then be looked for.

Long-standing symptoms

It's important that you mention to your doctor any long-standing symptoms – anything that appears to you as different from the norm, for some people have had fibromyalgia since childhood. If you always sensed something was wrong, felt you were different from others, here is your chance to put forward your case.

The examination

During the brief medical examination, your doctor will press firmly with a thumb on various parts of your body. People with fibromyalgia have areas of tenderness in specific locations, usually at junctions of muscle and bone. These 'tender points' are often exquisitely painful when pressed. Otherwise they may or may not be painful. As the degree of pressure used would not normally cause pain, it is a good, but not foolproof, indicator of the condition.

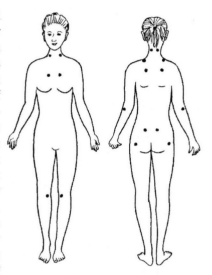

Figure 1 The 18 tender points used to establish a diagnosis of fibromyalgia

In 1990, the American College of Rheumatology defined the official criteria for the diagnosis of fibromyalgia. It is:

1 a history of pain in both sides of the body, pain above and below the waist, pain along the spine; and
2 pain or tenderness in 11 out of 18 tender points, sited at specific locations in the body (see Figure 1).

Myofascial pain syndrome

In many, the tender points are confined to one area of the body, such as around the shoulders or in the lower back. This indicates the presence of myofascial pain syndrome (known as MPS), a condition of localized severe chronic pain. In fact, the pain of MPS is often the worst part of fibromyalgia, as it is common for a person with fibromyalgia to also have MPS, particularly if their fibromyalgia was triggered by an injury. I have MPS in my upper back, shoulders and the base of my neck, which arose in the few years after my whiplash injury. It is the area of which I have to be most careful and which causes me the most difficulty.

Unfortunately, many doctors still fail to diagnose MPS.

Conditions similar to fibromyalgia

In some cases, tests are advised to rule out diseases with similar symptoms to fibromyalgia, such as arthritis, multiple sclerosis, lupus and an underactive thyroid gland.

I should add that until the diagnosis is made, it's common for people with fibromyalgia to worry that they are in the early stages of a more serious and perhaps terminal disease, such as cancer. Also, many start to wonder whether they are going mad. After all, it's not usual to hurt so much for no obvious reason and have a whole plethora of other mysterious ailments. It doesn't help that others may mistrust your assertions of pain and so on, and that even your doctor seems unsure of what's wrong. The fibromyalgia diagnosis comes as a terrific relief, therefore.

Your doctor

Fibromyalgia is not included in the National Institute for Health and Clinical Excellence (NICE) guidelines for recognized health conditions. As a result, some doctors still don't appreciate the complexities of the condition, or its many quirks. Fibromyalgia is now briefly described to students in medical school, but a doctor who left medical school before 1990 may not yet be familiar with it. That said, plenty of older doctors keep up to date with the latest medical news. In the end, the best doctor for you is the one who listens to you, works with you and offers the most useful treatments.

A rheumatologist

If your doctor is unable to make a definitive diagnosis, or your symptoms are not responding to conventional treatments, you may be referred to a rheumatologist at your local hospital's outpatient department. A rheumatologist is a specialist in disorders of the joints, muscles and other soft tissues.

After osteoarthritis, fibromyalgia is the second most common diagnosis made by rheumatologists. The condition therefore accounts for a large proportion of rheumatology outpatient visits. The usual age of fibromyalgia onset is between 30 and 60 years old, but it can develop at any age.

In the long term

Long-term rheumatology care has shown that it's unusual for people with fibromyalgia to develop another rheumatic disease or neurological condition. It is common, though, for a woman with fibromyalgia who is both very out of condition and post-menopausal to develop osteoporosis, which is a gradual weakening of the bones due to calcium loss.

If you think that you are at risk of osteoporosis, ask your doctor to refer you to a local hospital for a bone density scan. In cases of calcium loss – that is, where you already have osteoporosis or are at risk of getting it – good treatment is available, and will include vitamin D tablets which aid the delivery of calcium into the bones. You should also consume a high-calcium diet and take as much exercise as the climate and your condition allows. Being out in the sun helps, too, but of course this is limited by the good old British climate.

People who already have a well-established rheumatic condition such as arthritis, rheumatoid arthritis, lupus or Sjögren's syndrome may go on to develop fibromyalgia at some point, as discussed on page 5.

2

The role of neurotransmitters

The main function of the central nervous system (CNS for short) is to send information all over the body via a series of chemical hormones known as 'neurotransmitters'. In other words, neurotransmitters transfer information from one nerve cell to another. The information in question may simply be 'walk', 'chew', 'raise your arm' or 'smile'. Pain messages are also transferred in this way.

How pain is experienced

When an injury occurs, nerve cells in the skin and tissues quickly detect it and start a rapid chain of events. To be more precise, when you burn your hand, for example, certain hormonal neurotransmitters immediately communicate the information via nerve pathways to the spinal cord, which transmits the message to the brain. On being informed that an injury has occurred, the brain takes instant action. In this case it would tell you to remove your hand from the source of heat and run cold water over it. The response to pain seems instantaneous as it takes only a millisecond to do something about it, such as pulling away your hand.

In a healthy person, the pain stops as soon as an injury has healed. For the reasons described in this chapter, this doesn't always happen in a chronic pain condition.

Chronic pain and fibromyalgia

In fibromyalgia, neurotransmitter imbalances cause the muscle spasms and so on, which damage the soft tissues. The imbalances arise, in the first place, from a hypersensitive nervous system, a condition known as 'central sensitization'.

That all hormonal neurotransmitters are correctly balanced – that they are manufactured and secreted in the right quantities – is vital to optimum brain function and overall good health. When one or more is out of balance, functional impairment can occur.

In fact, neurotransmitter imbalance is thought to be the main reason for the whole gamut of symptoms in fibromyalgia. It is also believed to be the main cause of the condition. To date, researchers have found several neurotransmitter dysfunctions in fibromyalgia. They are now working on developing medications to address the problems.

Neurotransmitter levels can be affected by everyday things, such as some of the foods we eat, some of the drugs we are prescribed and even good old sunshine. In fibromyalgia, at least six neurotransmitters can be out of balance, meaning that their levels may be too high, too low or inefficiently manufactured and used by the body. Unfortunately, there is no clinical test available to measure neurotransmitter levels. Doctors have no choice but to assume that, in fibromyalgia, we all have similar neurotransmitter dysfunctions.

Nociceptors and central sensitization

The hypersensitive nervous system in fibromyalgia gives rise to irritation of the nerve endings responsible for sending pain signals (called 'nociceptors'). As a result, the nociceptors fail to receive sufficient oxygen, glucose and other nutrients, and their blood flow and energy production are severely disrupted. And the more irritated the nociceptors become, the more pain they produce. This creates the 'wind-up' situation known as central sensitization where the central nervous system is so highly sensitized, it sends out pain far too easily. In time, the spinal cord itself can become sensitized and transmit pain all over the body. The result is the widespread pain of fibromyalgia.

Neuropathic pain

Nociception, as described above, is one type of chronic pain. The other type is neuropathic pain, which occurs when the nerves of either the central or peripheral nervous system are actually damaged, maybe by the initial trauma that triggered fibromyalgia. Some people with fibromyalgia, including myself, have both types of chronic pain. In my case, damage to a disc in my lumbar (lower) spine causes it to compress my spinal cord and so send out pain. The damage arose in the first place when I walked up a very steep hill in cold weather when I wasn't too well. I now avoid putting myself in such risky situations.

Neurotransmitter pairs

The neurotransmitters involved in fibromyalgia come in pairs. They are:

- serotonin and melatonin
- norepinephrine and dopamine
- GABA and glutamate.

Serotonin and melatonin

The hormone serotonin is one of the major neurotransmitters in the body. Indeed, its manufacture, quantity and regulation play an important role in many of our bodily functions, including sleep, appetite, learning and pain perception. It is closely involved in determining our mood. Serotonin levels are, in fact, invariably very low in people who are depressed. Low serotonin is also a factor in obsessive–compulsive disorders (OCD), post-traumatic stress disorder (PTSD) and attention-deficit/hyperactivity disorder (ADHD).

If an individual is under a lot of emotional stress, their serotonin levels automatically drop. This is partly what makes fibromyalgia such a confounding disorder – we are stressed because we feel unwell and life has become limited, but the stress only goes to further reduce our serotonin levels and create further stress. It's a vicious circle that can be difficult, but not impossible, to break.

Serotonin is manufactured in the brain and gastrointestinal tract, travelling in chemical form along nerve pathways to perform particular functions. Neurotransmitters act together in complex networks, relaying a multitude of messages that prompt specific functions. The chief partner of serotonin is the chemical neurotransmitter melatonin. When levels of serotonin and melatonin are abnormally low, as is usually the case in fibromyalgia, the following symptoms can occur:

- feeling the cold
- hot flushes
- headaches
- appetite changes
- poor libido
- moodiness
- depression.

Extremely low serotonin levels can cause the following:

- muscle cramps
- bowel and bladder problems
- rapid, uncontrolled thinking
- emotional numbness
- emotional outbursts
- escape fantasies
- dwelling on traumatic experiences
- thoughts of self-harm or harming others.

The more of the above-mentioned symptoms you have, the lower your serotonin levels are likely to be. If you think that your serotonin levels may be extremely low but your doctor isn't aware of this, you need to seek urgent medical attention, making your symptoms very clear.

Chronic fatigue syndrome and serotonin

Chronic fatigue syndrome (CFS) is similar to fibromyalgia. However, pain is the main symptom in fibromyalgia and fatigue the main symptom in CFS. Many people have both syndromes – I do myself – but doctors don't always give two separate diagnoses. In fibromyalgia, serotonin levels are almost universally low, but experts have not yet clarified the matter with regard to CFS.

In CFS serotonin levels can be too high or too low, or they may be just right. Plenty of serotonin may be available for use, but research has indicated that the brain can fail to make use of it properly, because of inefficient receptors.

In the UK, CFS is commonly known as myalgic encephalomyelitis (ME).

The sleep cycle

Serotonin and melatonin are closely involved in the sleep cycle, serotonin being at its maximum when we are awake and at its minimum when we are asleep. When it gets dark in the evening, a certain amount of serotonin in the body is converted into melatonin, which helps us to fall asleep. And when light hits our eyelids in the morning, serotonin is released into our brains, helping us to wake up feeling refreshed and alert. The fibromyalgia-related shortfall of serotonin and melatonin is the main reason for the disturbed sleep patterns so characteristic of fibromyalgia. It is also the reason for our difficulty attaining deep sleep (stage 4 sleep), the state in which bodily tissues are regenerated and repaired. In addition, it may be the cause of the fatigue that is evident in so many, even after rest.

Serotonin levels in females

Research has shown that females are less able to produce serotonin than males. In fact, we normally have one-third less of the chemical in our bodies. This is probably the main reason why females are more susceptible to developing fibromyalgia. Up to 90 per cent of the fibromyalgia population is female.

Serotonin and sunlight

Exposure to sunlight is one of the best natural means of stimulating serotonin production in the body. It doesn't have to be warm sun, either – a sunny but cool winter's day should provide just as much of a serotonin boost. Serotonin stocks can even be replenished when sunlight is filtered by clouds.

Serotonin and pain

When we are hurting all the time, our bodies continue to manufacture serotonin. This is because serotonin is involved in pain regulation and the body perceives pain as a major threat to its well-being. A healthy person would find their serotonin levels automatically dropping to enable them to fall asleep, but this doesn't happen in chronic pain conditions where pain levels are constantly high. This is a major reason why sleep is so difficult to achieve in fibromyalgia.

So, if persistent pain makes the body produce a lot of serotonin, why aren't serotonin levels high instead of low in fibromyalgia? The answer is simply that our bodies battle hard to quell the pain, but they simply can't do it without help, since the underlying causes of the condition keep on producing more pain. It is only in successfully managing the pain that our bodies allow serotonin to improve our sleep.

Here are some brief recommendations for managing chronic pain (pain relief is the main focus of this book and will be discussed in greater detail in later pages):

- Take your prescribed medication.
- Distract yourself, for example by taking up absorbing hobbies.
- Use balms, creams, gels and lotions to ease localized pain.
- Use hot and cold therapy (see page 40), a TENS machine or pain pen (see page 33).

- Learn to handle stressful situations (see pages 38–41 and 90–4).
- Use pacing, take up a daily exercise regime, improve your diet, and adopt good posture (see Chapter 4).
- Learn how to relax and perform a daily relaxation routine.
- Take the recommended nutritional supplements and herbal remedies.

Dieting and serotonin production

Women are more likely than men to indulge in serotonin-depleting behaviour, such as going on a weight-loss diet. The fact is, though, that serotonin depends largely on carbohydrates for its many reactions in the body – known as 'synthesis'. In a diet, fats and proteins are often reduced too, yet these food groups are also involved in serotonin synthesis. A depletion of serotonin reserves can lead to strong food cravings and the desire to binge on something high-carb and/or high-fat. For instance, you might be unable to resist eating a full box of chocolates during a diet. Doing so would boost your serotonin levels and give you a temporary sense of well-being, and this would be followed by intense guilt – but you may not have had the craving in the first place if you were not restricting certain foods.

In fibromyalgia, it is advisable to eat a varied diet with appropriate amounts from all the food groups. Enjoy your food, don't hurry or overeat; and try to get plenty of rest and exercise every day. If you need to lose weight but are having trouble doing so, ask your doctor to refer you to a dietician who is well acquainted with fibromyalgia. If you are asked to cut down on carbs or fats, it would be best if you found another dietician.

Substance P

The normal pain process begins with the sudden rise in levels of a chemical neurotransmitter called 'substance P' in response to a painful stimulus such as a trapped finger or stubbed toe. Substance P uses nerve pathways to tell the brain to dilate blood cells in the injured area and perhaps cause some leakage of fluid and proteins from the cells involved. The effect is pain, swelling and inflammation.

The unusual thing about serotonin is that the lower its levels are, the more substance P is pumped into the body. In fact, scientific research has shown conclusively that substance P levels are around three times higher in fibromyalgia than they should be. This causes us to be much more sensitive to pain than the average person. Other chronic pain disorders display slight elevations of substance P, but in no other condition are the levels nearly so high as in fibromyalgia.

When levels of substance P are significantly raised, as in fibromyalgia, the substance is likely to spill over from injured tissues to neighbouring healthy tissues, increasing, in turn, their sensitivity to pain. In some instances, the chemical pervades the entire spinal cord, causing sensitization of all the bodily tissues and making everyday activities result in pain. After doing something so seemingly insignificant as scratching a tiny itch, many people with fibromyalgia – myself included – experience acute pain in that area, lasting for several minutes. Some people are so sensitized to pain that they have no choice but to do very little. As a consequence, they become very weak, which further depletes their serotonin levels and raises substance P.

I found myself in this dire situation in the early days of my illness. I became so weak and pain-sensitive that I was bed-bound for 16 long months. So how did I come to write 20 books and be able to take four-mile walks? Well, serotonin supplementation in the form of drugs improved my condition to some extent (see Chapter 3), but my main saviour was, to start with, performing one or two stretching exercises each day. Tentative strengthening exercises followed and in time I was able to sit up for a while. It took a couple of years for me to be well enough to begin really enjoying my life again, but my persistence during that period was well worth while.

As well as low serotonin and high substance P levels, research has shown that some of us have decreased blood flow to certain areas of the brain. These are believed to be the areas that help to modulate transmitted pain signals. Whether this problem occurs prior to the onset of fibromyalgia or as a result of it is not yet known. Research is ongoing in this respect.

How you can increase serotonin levels

Since a shortfall of serotonin provokes high substance P levels, it makes sense to say that increasing levels of available serotonin and improving the ability of the body to use it should reduce many fibromyalgia symptoms, including the pain. Serotonin levels can be boosted naturally by exposure to sunshine, but sunshine isn't always around – far from it. It is believed that eating certain foods can also help, but this is far from certain.

Serotonin-enhancing foods

There is a theory, supported by some studies, that eating a certain diet can enhance serotonin levels. What is not known is whether the filter we all have that allows only certain substances through to the brain – called the 'blood–brain barrier' – is sufficiently penetrated by the foods in question to have an effect. Much more research is required in this area to prove whether or not there is a link between certain foods and raised serotonin levels.

Foods that are commonly believed to contain building blocks of serotonin, and therefore raise levels of serotonin in your blood, include grains, beans, dark chocolate and watermelon (the latter only considered healthy in small amounts). In order to make more serotonin available to your brain, you may prefer to try the recommended nutritional supplements before thinking of using drug therapy. See pages 99–102 and Chapter 6 for more information.

Drugs that improve neurotransmitter activity

When fibromyalgia first came to light as a disorder of significance, the pain was thought to originate from the body's periphery – the muscles, tendons and ligaments. There are certainly problems in peripheral areas in fibromyalgia; however, they are now believed to originate from neurotransmitter errors. Indeed, the reason that some of us are sensitive all over is that the neurotransmitter substance P can spill over into healthy tissues, as already discussed.

This section describes the drugs aimed at treating central nervous system problems.

Tricyclic antidepressants

As with all the antidepressant medications used in fibromyalgia, tricyclic antidepressants are not taken specifically to treat depression, but are used to tackle the pain, fatigue, sleep problems and so on. Moreover, they must be taken in smaller amounts than required for depression alone. The depression often tied in with fibromyalgia usually arises from the twofold problems of neurotransmitter dysfunction and the stresses of living with a painful condition. It is known as 'reactive depression'.

Tricyclics include Elavil (amitriptyline), Elronon (nortriptyline), Tofranil (imipramine) and Evadyne (butriptyline), and they act by blocking the re-uptake of both serotonin and norepinephrine. Because the newer antidepressants (see below) have fewer side effects, tricyclics have largely been replaced in clinical use. The primary side effects associated with tricyclics include dry mouth, drowsiness, nausea, dizziness, constipation, morning 'hangover', disturbed sleep, weight gain and sometimes anxiety. As tricyclics have sedative qualities, they are best taken an hour or so before bedtime.

Selective serotonin re-uptake inhibitors (SSRIs)

If you have had fibromyalgia for a while, you are likely to have heard of selective serotonin re-uptake inhibitors (SSRIs), the most common of which are Prozac (fluoxetine), Paxil (paroxetine), Serzone (nefazodone hydrochloride) and Zoloft (sertraline). Serotonin is released by particular nerve cells and later reabsorbed back into the same cells in a natural cleaning-up process. SSRIs effectively slow this cleaning-up process, keeping the serotonin around for longer to help improve pain, fatigue, cognitive impairment, depression and sleep.

As serotonin is required in adequate quantities to improve pain, sleep and other fibromyalgia-related problems, it would seem sensible to say that keeping more of it around in the body should greatly improve matters. It's an unfortunate fact, though, that SSRIs often fail. Indeed, blocking the re-uptake of serotonin doesn't do a lot of good if there is very little serotonin around in the first place.

SSRIs are not addictive, but their associated side effects include a risk of nervousness, dry mouth, headache, nausea, diarrhoea, loss of appetite, weight loss and problems with sleeping. They may also cause drowsiness, headache, fatigue, nausea, vomiting and reduced libido. If you are thinking of taking SSRIs, be aware of the possible side effects; and inform your doctor if the side effects are in any way intolerable. Most people with fibromyalgia will try several prescription antidepressants (such as SSRIs, SNRIs, tricyclics and so on), yet often no significant benefit is obtained. Strangely, the newer and supposedly more potent SSRIs such as Cipramil (citalopram) appear to be less effective than the older types.

If you want to stop using SSRIs – either due to side effects or to assess your condition when you are not taking them – be aware that abrupt discontinuation can lead to withdrawal symptoms in the form of anxiety, moodiness, trembling and so on. Your doctor will be able to guide you through a gradual reduction in the dosage. Once your system is clear of them, you may realize that they were in fact helping you, in which case you can start taking them again, gradually building up the dosage. The opposite might become apparent, however, and you find that they were not helping at all, in which case you are better off without the type you were taking.

Selective norepinephrine re-uptake inhibitors (SNRIs)

SNRIs are a fairly new type of drug, but may already be the most widely used antidepressant today. They work in the same way as SSRIs, except that they inhibit the reabsorption of norepinephrine as well as serotonin (norepinephrine is yet another neurotransmitter involved in determining pain levels, sleep quality and so on). People with fibromyalgia have a shortfall of norepinephrine as well as serotonin, and the double inhibition is often better at reducing symptoms. Indeed, recent studies have indicated that for some people the combination of serotonin and norepinephrine re-uptake inhibition has stronger analgesic effects than substances that inhibit the re-uptake of either neurotransmitter alone.

Norepinephrine is also important because our bodies use it to produce dopamine, and since norepinephrine is in low supply in fibromyalgia, so is dopamine (see pages 20–1 for information on dopamine). The symptoms related to low dopamine include difficulty concentrating, muscle aches, tremor, impaired fine motor skills and poor coordination. The symptoms related to low norepinephrine include loss of alertness, decreased libido, memory problems and depression. As SNRIs work in a similar way to SSRIs, they have side effects in common. However, the side effects are often milder and therefore more tolerable. As a result, SNRIs are now the antidepressants of choice.

As with any drug, you will only find out whether SNRIs will work for you by giving them a try. Using a diary to record how you are feeling every day can make improvements more apparent than if you simply try to remember how you were before you began taking them.

Note that many drugs, antidepressants included, can work better in the early days or months of their use. As we don't know whether, or when, a drug's ability to help will at some point start to falter, try to make good use of the possible 'window of opportunity' by eating healthily and getting as much exercise as you can to build up your strength. Exercise should always be careful and interspersed with sensible rest periods.

Examples of SNRIs are Cymbalta (duloxetine), Savella (milnacipran), Effexor (venlafaxine) and Pristiq (desvenlafaxine). A recent analysis of clinical trials into duloxetine, taken at 60mg daily, showed that it significantly reduced pain in more than half of the patients treated – women, in this case, as women respond better to the drug because of hormonal differences between the sexes. The drug was also found to benefit fatigue, as well as physical and mental performance. The improvement in pain intensity levelled off after about three months, however. Duloxetine should not be taken if you abuse alcohol or have chronic liver disease.

Milnacipran has been shown in studies to be the most effective SNRI for treating fibromyalgia. Indeed, data collected from several recent double-blind placebo controlled trials have suggested that fibromyalgia volunteers taking 100mg or 200mg milnacipran daily were very much improved with respect to pain and physical function. A large clinical trial of milnacipran in fibromyalgia patients who were unresponsive to duloxetine is currently under way. When milnacipran works, it is as effective in men as it is in women. Start with a low dose, say 50g, and gradually build up to 100g daily. If your symptoms don't improve, it can be increased as high as 200g.

Sudden discontinuation of SNRIs will usually prompt withdrawal symptoms (as with SSRIs). If you wish to stop taking them, gradually reduce them under your doctor's watchful eye.

Norepinephrine and dopamine

Norepinephrine converts into dopamine in the brain, so low norepinephrine levels means low dopamine levels. The chief aims of dopamine are to aid concentration and help control how your body moves. Low dopamine levels are associated with difficulty concentrating, memory problems, inability to focus and stiff, achy muscles. In more severe cases, low dopamine can result in tremor, impaired fine motor skills, poor balance and coordination, and strange walking gait.

People with fibromyalgia are likely to be deficient in dopamine. Indeed, this is thought to be the main reason for our cognitive problems – poor memory, difficulty concentrating, word mix-ups and so on. Low dopamine can even be the cause of the tremors, and coordination and balance problems experienced by some people with fibromyalgia.

Unfortunately, SNRIs sometimes raise the levels of serotonin and dopamine too much. Excess dopamine in the body can cause psychological disturbances, such as euphoria, suspicion, excessive focus, and difficulty judging what is important from what isn't. If you have any of these symptoms, you should visit your doctor straight away.

Drugs that increase the availability of dopamine

If you have one or more of the symptoms linked to low dopamine levels, you may find SNRI drugs useful. If they fail to really help, your doctor may be able to redress the balance, at least partly, by recommending a dopamine stimulant. Such drugs belong to the methylphenidate family and include Ritalin, Concerta and Methadate.

Dopamine-enhancing foods

Although there is some clinical evidence that certain foods can elevate dopamine levels – chicken, wheat germ, fish, cheese, eggs, apples, bananas, watermelon, beetroot, beans, legumes, blueberry extract, red wine, green tea and black tea – you would probably need to devour ridiculous amounts to achieve the desired result. No harm can come, though, from adding these highly nutritious foods to a healthy balanced diet.

Nutritional supplements that increase dopamine

Since SNRIs can only inhibit whatever quantity of norepinephrine is actually available in our bodies, we really need to look for other means of boosting its levels and so of increasing dopamine. The following are believed to help:

- Beta-nicotinamide adenine dinucleotide (NADH) – a natural co-enzyme, available in supplement form
- L-theanine – an amino acid found only in green and black tea
- Omega 3 fatty acids – fish oil capsules or flax oil
- Rhodiola rosea – an adaptogenic herb.

See pages 107–8 for more information about these particular substances.

GABA and glutamate

You may have heard a lot about serotonin and dopamine, but very little about GABA and glutamate; yet they are all fellow neurotransmitters, and all vitally important. The brain uses glutamate to produce GABA, but in fibromyalgia the conversion process is somehow faulty. This makes two further dysfunctional neurotransmitters.

Glutamate has a stimulatory effect on the brain; it gets us fired up, excited, ready for action. The trouble is, it sometimes doesn't know how far to go and keeps on pumping up the neurons (the cells that transfer nerve messages) until, no longer able to cope with the excitement, they give in and die. Glutamate is therefore known as an 'excitotoxin' and is believed to be involved in degenerative brain conditions such as Alzheimer's disease.

Low levels of GABA

Just as the pairings serotonin and melatonin, and norepinephrine and dopamine, work together to create a particular effect, so the neurotransmitters glutamate and GABA have a close working relationship. GABA stands for gamma-amino-n-butyric acid, and it is classed as an 'inhibitory neurotransmitter' because its chief function is to calm the brain. It is therefore involved in sleep, relaxation, anxiety regulation and muscle performance. Disorders such as chronic anxiety, depression and chronic muscle tension are related to impairment in GABA performance.

Although a synthetic form of GABA is available as a supplement, many experts believe that it would not effectively cross the blood–brain barrier – the protective barrier we all have to prevent damaging substances from entering the circulatory system supplying the brain. Other experts, however, are of the opinion that high doses of GABA would allow some of it to cross. Clearly, much more research is required to clarify the situation.

When GABA levels are either too low or performing inefficiently, glutamate takes precedence. As a result, the neurons are very easily overexcited and may die. Inefficient GABA production gives rise to anxiety disorders such as panic attacks, seizure disorders, addictions, headaches and cognitive impairment. As caffeine has been shown to drastically inhibit the release of GABA, a good way of knowing what having low GABA feels like is to remember what it feels like to have drunk too much coffee – it makes your brain race and you feel edgy for a while.

Even though plenty of websites and health food shops sell GABA, there is a noticeable shortfall of scientific evidence to support the manufacturers' many claims. As the side effects include raised insulin production, it would clearly be a problem for people with hyperinsulinaemia and syndrome X, both of which are pre-diabetic states. Some people have reported anxiety attacks, tingling and nausea after taking a dose of GABA, yet many experience no side effects at all.

Tranquillizing drugs such as the benzodiazepines and barbiturates work by increasing or imitating the effect of GABA.

Brain excitability due to raised glutamate levels

Interestingly, in 2008, US researchers found that the pain of volunteer fibromyalgia patients decreased when their glutamate levels were low.[1] Researchers had previously suspected that glutamate was involved in chronic pain conditions, since earlier studies had shown that some areas of the brain are highly excited in fibromyalgia. More recent trials using a brain imaging technique known as 'proton magnetic resonance spectroscopy' (H-MRS) have demonstrated that glutamate levels drop when pain levels are reduced by natural means, such as acupuncture, aromatherapy massage and warm baths, and so on. It is suspected that the drop is only temporary, however, since such treatments have only a short-lived effect.

It makes sense to say, then, that taking steps to reduce your pain levels naturally and consistently – for example, by using complementary therapies, getting regular exercise, improving your diet, avoiding overexertion and being careful to pace yourself – should effectively lower your glutamate levels and keep them down, reducing the excitability of your brain and generally improving your condition. The main focus of this book is on pain-lowering techniques.

Experts believe that in the future the severity of fibromyalgia could be assessed by measuring glutamate levels.

Human growth hormone

As if the errors found in three pairs of neurotransmitters weren't enough, there is also a dysfunction in human growth hormone

(HGH) in fibromyalgia. In fact, studies published some 25 years ago suggested that getting extra GABA into the brain can increase HGH by a massive amount (up to 500 per cent). Later studies, in which fibromyalgia volunteers were given hormone injection therapy, have indicated the same positive outcome, the volunteers reporting less muscle weakness and morning stiffness, and a reduced number of tender points.

One very rigidly controlled study in 2003 of body builders and GABA has thrown doubt on the whole matter, though.[2] When the hormone was taken prior to exercise, HGH levels increased, but when taken at other times of the day (not before exercise), there was no change. As it is body builders we are talking about, be clear that the exercise took the form of a strenuous physical workout. All in all, it appears that GABA is capable of raising HGH levels and that some of it must cross the blood–brain barrier, but possibly only after exercise or exertion. A 2007 review of all the literature on the matter reported a need for further study before any solid recommendations can be made.

Although some pharmacies and health shops sell HGH formulas, you really should seek your doctor's advice. HGH is available in limited quantities to some fibromyalgia patients.

3

Medications for pain

The chief problem in fibromyalgia is how to manage the pain. It's a vexation with which we are faced every hour of every day. We spend a lot of money on natural remedies, only to find most of them less than satisfactory; we try over-the-counter painkillers, but for many they're not powerful enough, so we weep in our doctor's office, and beg for something stronger, something that will make a real difference. The doctor prescribes long-term medication in the form of antidepressants (for pain, not depression, in fibromyalgia) or anticonvulsants (for their pain-lowering properties), and these may improve matters to a degree, but they seldom stop symptom flare-ups where the pain can be all-consuming, where it sends you to bed for days, weeks or even months, just waiting for the time when you can get up again. On top of that, flare-ups are weakening; they make us more prone to accidentally overdoing it. And so the cycle continues . . .

It's possible to live a decent life with low levels of pain, using natural techniques and painkillers as required. Higher pain levels make getting on with things very difficult. Indeed, we really need stronger drugs to reduce how much we hurt, so that it settles at a tolerable level. Unfortunately, when insufficient action is taken to reduce severe pain, neurotransmitter levels can shift further out of balance and prompt a further increase in pain (there is no upper limit to pain intensity). Neurotransmitter dysfunctions can also make restful sleep impossible, causing us to wake up unrefreshed, with stiff muscles and low mood.

The long-term medications for fibromyalgia are often aimed at balancing certain neurotransmitter levels. When this is achieved, symptoms can greatly improve. Not all long-term medications are effective, however, and many create intolerable side effects. Moreover, lots of people with fibromyalgia have sensitivity reactions to chemical medications. If you tend to react badly to new medications, ask your doctor to start you on the lowest dosage. In this way, you can slowly build up to the recommended dosage with less risk of problems. If, in time, the drug stops having a positive effect (the state of 'tolerance'), inform your doctor and with his or her support slowly stop taking it. You'll find that some drugs don't seem to work for you at all, whereas others make you feel much improved. If you are taking a new medication but see no positive results after three months, there's no point in continuing to take it. You will still need to come off the drug very slowly.

Until the last few years, there was very little research into the best medications for fibromyalgia. I am pleased to report, though, that researchers are now looking into the peculiarities of fibromyalgia and we hope to have much better drug treatment in the coming months and years.

Painkillers (analgesics)

Painkillers are medications designed to 'take the edge off' pain and, in fibromyalgia, to combat flare-ups. They work mainly by interfering with the pain signals going to and coming from the brain, but can also change the way the brain interprets pain signals, with the same pain-reducing effect.

Painkillers are available over the counter in pharmacies, or from your doctor on prescription. The over-the-counter painkiller most commonly used in fibromyalgia is paracetamol (in the USA this is known as Tylenol (acetaminophen)). This drug has analgesic properties similar to aspirin, but is generally tolerated better. The possible side effects linked to paracetamol are feverishness, bleeding or bruising, sore mouth and lips, rashes or hives, a stabbing pain in the lower back or side and unexplained weakness. If you experience any of these problems, it's important that you see your doctor.

Unfortunately, paracetamol is not capable of providing the efficient, long-term relief required in fibromyalgia. The drug may benefit headaches, achiness and non-severe pain, but you may need something stronger for more radical relief.

Paracetamol is now often combined with an opioid analgesic (see pages 28–9) to tackle severe chronic pain, but the dosage must be increased very gradually to reduce the risk of side effects (nausea, vomiting, drowsiness, dry mouth, urinary retention, constipation and sudden drop in blood pressure on standing up). Although fears of addiction are still associated with long-term opioid intake, most experts are convinced that these fears are unfounded. They even assert that such drugs can be taken safely for years, providing continuous satisfactory relief.

Anti-inflammatory medications

Two types of anti-inflammatory drug are used in fibromyalgia – the traditional non-steroidal anti-inflammatory drug (NSAID) and the newer Cox-II inhibitor drug. Although fibromyalgia is not truly an inflammatory condition, certain nerve endings are often inflamed. In addition, we sometimes have secondary problems, such as inflammation of the wrist, elbow, shoulder and knee (known commonly as tendonitis, tennis elbow, frozen shoulder and housemaid's knee). In some cases, flare-ups respond well to anti-inflammatory drugs, too.

Non-steroidal anti-inflammatory drugs (NSAIDs)

NSAIDs work by inhibiting the production of a substance in the body called the Cox enzyme, thus reducing the number of pain-creating chemicals called prostaglandins. The NSAIDs available on prescription include Advil (ibuprofen), Indocin (indomethacin), Naprosyn/Aleve (naproxen), Voltaren (diclofenac), Relafen (nabumetone), Feldene (piroxicam) and Lodine (etodolac). Aspirin is also an NSAID and can be purchased over the counter.

Low dosage ibuprofen is available over the counter, but you will need a doctor's prescription to secure a higher dosage. However, you should not take over-the-counter ibuprofen for more than ten days without your doctor's consent, and it can interact with other drugs, such as those for high blood pressure (hypertension). As ibuprofen thins the blood, patients on warfarin should also be careful to avoid it. Until research is carried out into the effects of NSAIDs on pregnancy, pregnant women should not take ibuprofen either.

The possible side effects linked to NSAIDs are diarrhoea, constipation, dizziness, rashes and headache. To reduce the possibility of gastrointestinal problems, NSAIDs should be taken with food. Long-term use requires close monitoring, as prolonged inhibition of prostaglandins can cause acid to seep through the stomach lining, resulting in gastrointestinal bleeding. Research has also indicated that NSAIDs can wreak havoc with vitamin stores in the body, which may contribute to fatigue. It is recommended, therefore, that NSAIDs are taken for a limited period only.

The effectiveness of NSAIDs varies from person to person. It appears that they can successfully reduce mild to moderate pain, but have little effect on severe pain. Their effect is relatively short-lived, too.

Cox-II inhibitors

Cox-II inhibitors are a new generation of anti-inflammatory drugs. They were developed as an alternative to NSAIDs, but with fewer undesirable side effects. The Cox-II inhibitors now available include Celebrex (celecoxib), Vioxx (rofecoxib) and the latest addition, Bextra (valdecoxib). They work by blocking the enzymes (known as Cox-II) responsible for causing stomach irritation and gastrointestinal problems. Interestingly, researchers now suspect that they also reduce hypersensitivity of the central nervous system (known as central sensitization). Further research is required to prove or disprove the matter.

Note that people with a history of heart (cardiovascular) disease should not take Vioxx as it can increase the risk of cardiovascular problems.

Narcotic analgesia

Narcotic analgesia in the form of opiates and opioids (the latter being derivatives of opiates) have long been around and are more commonly known as codeine and morphine. Many doctors are wary of prescribing narcotics, though, and they may only be offered in a hospital setting or in life-limiting conditions. The vast majority of fibromyalgia patients can manage without such strong painkillers, but studies have shown that they can make a great difference for severe symptoms, providing longer relief and allowing the individual to get much more from their life.

It's a shame that some doctors still insist that narcotics are not appropriate for chronic pain. They fear that long-term use would have the same effect as if they were taken by a healthy person – that addiction would occur. They also fear that the person would need increasingly higher doses to achieve the same pain-relieving effect – the situation known as 'tolerance'. All the long-term studies into narcotics and chronic pain disorders have shown a positive outcome, however, for it seems that drugs taken for pain seldom hit the 'pleasure centres' of the brain. Indeed, the vast majority of volunteer pain patients in the studies mentioned experienced long-term relief with no need to increase the dosage, and only a tiny minority, 0.5 per cent of them, showed any sign of addiction – that's one person in every 200. I would imagine that those particular individuals had only a mild case of fibromyalgia.

Antidepressants

Neurotransmitter-altering medications are known generally as antidepressants. When this family of drugs is prescribed in fibromyalgia to reduce pain levels, they are required in a lower dosage than when used for depression alone.

The antidepressants used in fibromyalgia are tricyclic antidepressants, SSRIs (selective serotonin reuptake inhibitors), and SNRIs (selective norepinephrine reuptake inhibitors). See pages 17–20 for information about antidepressants.

Muscle relaxants

Muscle relaxants appear to act on the central nervous system and are often taken to ease tight, tense muscles and muscles in spasm. Unfortunately, though, they are said to be no more effective than paracetamol in this respect. Sleep can be greatly improved by muscle relaxants, but because of their propensity for creating dependence, it can be more and more difficult to sleep without them. They are therefore mostly prescribed at a low dosage to help you over a sleepless period. Rather than taking muscle relaxants during the night, it is best to take them shortly before you go to bed, so they don't cause drowsiness the next morning when you may have to drive.

Muscle relaxants include Valium (diazepam), Soma (carisprodol) and Flexeril (cyclobenzaprine hydrochloride). They are not among the 'first-line' agents in fibromyalgia, but are sometimes turned to when all else has failed. There is actually a small amount of evidence, from a 2005 clinical review, that muscle relaxants can boost the function of NSAIDs.[3] Further research into this matter is clearly needed.

As well as drowsiness and sedation, the other side effects linked to muscle relaxants are dry mouth, constipation, headache, heart palpitations, urinary retention and reactions with other medications. People who suffer depression or have a history of drug or alcohol addiction should not be prescribed muscle relaxants.

Antispastic medications

Although antispastic medications were designed to ease the muscle spasm linked to multiple sclerosis, cerebral palsy and certain spinal injuries, they are now known to benefit fibromyalgia, too. The two main antispastic medications are Zanaflex (tizanidine) and Baclofen (lioresal). Zanaflex can inhibit the action of the pain-transmitting hormone substance P (levels of which are at least three times greater than normal in people with fibromyalgia), limiting the number of pain messages it can send to the brain. The drug appears to be well tolerated and often significantly lowers substance P levels, improving sleep, pain and physical function. Levels of a chemical called transaminase (this appears naturally in our bodies) should be monitored during treatment with Zanaflex.

Baclofen effectively activates the GABA receptor (see pages 22–4 for information on the neurotransmitter GABA), which often results in the general relaxation of tense and tight muscles. A very positive property of Baclofen is that it doesn't create tolerance. In other words, it should retain its anti-spasmodic effects after many years of use. In a few cases, extreme drowsiness can occur, but most escape this.

Anticonvulsants

Anticonvulsant (anti-seizure) medications were originally designed for the treatment of epilepsy, a neurological disorder marked by convulsions. Medical professionals soon found, though, that this type of drug could help people with fibromyalgia, especially those with neuropathic pain – burning, electric shock-like feelings caused by nerve irritation. The possible side effects associated with anticonvulsants include drowsiness, dry mouth, constipation, nausea, vomiting, blurred vision, weight gain, dizziness and cognitive problems (confusion, poor memory and difficulty concentrating). In some cases, the cognitive problems are so severe that it is impossible to continue taking the drug.

The anticonvulsants most commonly prescribed are Lyrica (pregabalin), Neurontin (gabapentin), Dilantin (phenytoin), Depakote (divalproex) and Tegretol (carbamazepine). Lyrica (pregabalin), however, is the anticonvulsant of choice at present. In a review of all the research into this drug, 40 per cent of people with fibromyalgia who used it felt 'very much improved'. If you are taking an anticonvulsant, your doctor should closely monitor your blood count and liver function as these can be affected by this type of drug.

I myself am unable to tolerate either Lyrica or Neurontin. Each of them drastically worsened my short-term memory and powers of concentration. I now steer clear of drugs in the anticonvulsant group, and recommend that you watch out for cognitive problems.

Trigger point injections

People with fibromyalgia usually have trigger points, these being areas of acute sensitivity located at the centre of ragged bands of taut muscle. When 'activated' by overwork, cold weather, stress and so on, a trigger point will radiate pain to further areas. When trigger points in one area are regularly activated, the problem is myofascial pain syndrome (as mentioned on page 7). MPS often develops in conjunction with fibromyalgia. It gives rise to the localized and often severe pain that, for those affected, is normally the worst part of fibromyalgia.

The best treatment of MPS is trigger point massage and manipulation. Unfortunately, to date, few physiotherapists are trained to do this. If you would like to try releasing your own trigger points, there are publications available giving information about this, such as the very helpful *The Trigger Point Therapy Workbook* (see Further reading at the back of this book).

On a short-term basis, trigger points respond well to heat treatments and sometimes acupuncture. Another option is to have trigger point injections, usually of local anaesthetic (lignocaine and its derivatives are most effective) combined with a corticosteroid. Trigger point injections, which work by breaking the cycle of pain within the tissues, should be administered only by a pain specialist familiar with the fibromyalgia condition. The actual location of the injection – whether or not it directly hits the troublesome spot – determines the level of pain relief. Dry needling – the insertion of a needle into the area without also injecting a medication – can be enough to break the pain cycle, but most specialists prefer to give their patient the optimum chance by injecting anaesthetic and a corticosteroid.

During or after a course of trigger point injections, you can improve your muscle tone by introducing gentle exercise; if you are already used to doing an exercise regime, this is the time to very gradually increase your repertoire. The injection acts for an average of three weeks. However, continued deactivation of the treated trigger points depends upon whether you can successfully improve your muscle tone during that time.

Botox injections

A small number of doctors are now injecting Botox into painful tissues to decrease muscle spasm. Botox is a form of botulinum poison commonly used in 'cosmetic fashion' to freeze-relax wrinkles and so smooth them out. However, since Botox has only a temporary effect and is costly, it is unlikely ever to be a favourite painkilling treatment.

Prolotherapy

In prolotherapy, a solution of sugar and water is injected into an area weakened by prolonged muscle spasm. The area becomes inflamed, blood supply increases and nutrients enter to stimulate the tissue. As a result, the soft tissues in the area, inclusive of tendons and ligaments, are encouraged to heal. The body should also make new cells in the area. A series of injections every few weeks is normally required for the optimum outcome. This safe and effective therapy is used in numerous pain conditions, but fibromyalgia pain from an unresolved whiplash injury responds best of all.

Guaifenesin

For several years, this over-the-counter cough and cold preparation has been promoted by Dr R. Paul St Amand for the treatment of fibromyalgia. He believes that we have an excess of phosphate in our cells which disrupts the way our muscles function, causing spasm and pain. He recommends the 'Guaifenesin Protocol' in tablet form to help excrete the excess phosphate in our urine.

However, in the only scientifically controlled study of fibromyalgia subjects, there was no real difference between the group taking a placebo and the group taking guaifenesin. It was concluded, then, that any improvement reported was due to the 'placebo effect', where the person's belief in a medication is so strong that they actually do feel better for a while. Still, Dr St Amand professes to have seen great success in his patients. He says that the study was flawed because some of the subjects were also taking aspirin, in a compound that may reduce the effectiveness of guaifenesin. Clearly, further research is required.

The TENS machine

A transcutaneous electrical nerve stimulator (TENS) machine produces a tingling/pulsating sensation as it transmits electrical impulses to the person's central nervous system (CNS). The impulses effectively block the sensation of pain in some cases. The small battery-operated devices are side effect free and easily attached to the waistband of a skirt or trousers. TENS machines can be worn the whole day, from early morning until bedtime, but you may need to use it for an hour or so before noticing any benefit.

Those who are lucky enough to experience relief from their TENS machines daily may be able to eliminate drugs entirely. However, many find that although the device works well at first, it becomes less effective after a few weeks, probably because the CNS learns to override the effects of repeated interference. Researchers are currently developing devices that overcome this problem by randomly switching stimulation on and off. In the meantime, using the machine for maybe two hours, then turning it off for two hours, can prolong its usefulness.

TENS machines can be purchased from certain pharmacies. You can also buy Purevive water-based gel to use with your TENS machine electrodes, to ease any irritation.

The pain pen

Many pharmacies also stock the pain pen – a small pen-like device which, when you press the 'clicker' at the top, delivers tiny electrical impulses. These impulses are believed to stimulate the brain to produce endorphins, the body's natural painkillers. The pen can be used directly at the site of pain, or at acupuncture sites, where it is said to be slightly more effective.

The pain pen is accompanied by a chart that shows which parts of the body require stimulation for pain relief in specific areas. When treating a migraine or headache, for example, stimulation must be applied to the opposite side of the body. So with a left-sided migraine you should click the pen (20–25 times) on the right side of the body, at the sites indicated on the chart.

This treatment is side effect free and fairly effective.

Interesting new developments

Although scientists have not yet uncovered the real nature of the 'insult' that gives rise to fibromyalgia, scientific advances are taking place all the time. New treatments for chronic illness are regularly being developed and tested, and I firmly believe that one day a pill that we can pop into our mouths will enable us to work our way back to full health. As yet, though, there is no one simple cure for fibromyalgia and we must ourselves try our utmost to work for improvements. This section discusses the promising new developments of today.

Cannabinoids

Cannabis, the most widely used illegal recreational drug in the UK, contains an active ingredient called tetrahydrocannabinol (THC), and it is this that makes a person happy, 'chilled out' or just sleepy. THC can also alter a person's sense of reality, causing them to see, hear or feel differently from normal and sometimes triggering mild hallucinations. It can release inhibitions, making people talkative, giggly and generally more animated. However, when taken regularly over a long period, there can be unwelcome effects – chronic anxiety, memory impairment and even long-term mental health problems such as depression and paranoia.

Why do I mention an illegal drug in a fibromyalgia book? Well, there is scientific evidence that cannabis or its derivatives may be useful as a medical treatment. In conditions with an element of pain, such as multiple sclerosis and muscular dystrophy, some patients smoke cannabis on a regular basis. The pain relief experienced is usually fairly mild, but often sufficient, especially when combined with its relaxing effect. Unfortunately, though, most people with fibromyalgia wouldn't obtain enough pain relief to make the procedure worthwhile. Moreover, cannabis is expensive and difficult to access.

The complex nature of the chemicals (known scientifically as cannabinoids) contained in the cannabis plant has made their scientific study very difficult. Now, though, they are all gradually being identified in large trials, which are also testing the safety and efficacy of synthetic cannabis extracts. So far it has been seen that several medical conditions should benefit from appropriate cannabinoid treatment. It seems that many people with fibromyalgia would benefit from cannabinoid therapy, with the exception of those with more severe symptoms. There is now also strong laboratory evidence that neuropathic pain (see page 11) can be calmed significantly by 'cannabinoid analgesia', when this is taken regularly. It is hoped that we won't have long to wait before cannabinoid analgesia is widely accessible, fully legal and available on prescription.

EEG-based stimulation

I was very interested to read in scientific literature that sometimes a whiplash injury can injure the brain and central nervous system, and that when this occurs a condition called 'EEG slowing' is likely to arise (even slight damage usually causes a slowing in brainwave activity) – the result of this being a greater risk of developing fibromyalgia. This is apparently the reason why a large number of fibromyalgia cases have a whiplash injury in common.

Now, electroencephalogram (EEG) technology can identify areas of the brain that are injured and functioning abnormally and EEG-based stimulation aimed at normalizing brainwave patterns can be given – although this therapy is not yet readily available. To help retrain the muscles, a treatment called surface electromyography (sEMG) will later be carried out, after which the person must work hard at improving their strength and mobility.

EEG-based stimulation is promising and we look forward to the day when it is widely available.

Growth hormone

Studies have shown that in fibromyalgia and chronic fatigue syndrome (CFS) there are abnormally low levels of a substance called IGF-1 (somatomedin-C), which is symbolic of inadequate growth hormone release. IGF-1 is mainly produced during deep sleep (stage 4 sleep), which means that a good night's sleep (and afternoon naps that don't keep you awake half the night) are essential to growth hormone release. IGF-1 is also produced during exercise, which is why exercise can make you feel better for a while. People with fibromyalgia and CFS almost always have IGF-1, and therefore growth hormone, in short supply.

Because research has shown that growth hormone supplementation has a rejuvenating effect on muscle cells, giving them more flexibility, strength and endurance, it should be useful in the treatment of fibromyalgia and CFS. So far, however, owing to its high cost and poor availability, it has been prescribed only to children who need to boost their height, while people with fibromyalgia and CFS have been denied it. There are indications that the situation may change before too long, and we do hope this happens. It's a shame that a treatment so conceivably useful to us should be withheld.

Growth hormone is produced in the body with the help of the hormone GABA (as discussed on pages 22–4).

Normast

Since 2010 there has been an exciting new painkiller on the scene called Normast, which has been hailed as a breakthrough in safe and effective chronic pain treatment. You don't even need a doctor's prescription to obtain it. The active ingredient in Normast is palmitoylethanolamide (PEA), a substance produced by the body's own cells and so present naturally as a fatty acid. Research has shown that Normast is capable of activating the body's own healing systems and can make a real difference in chronic conditions such as neuropathic pain, sciatica, multiple sclerosis pain, diabetic neuropathy, prostate pain, pelvic pain, carpal tunnel pain, lumbosacral pain and the pain after stroke.

Because Normast is a natural substance, it is registered as a food for medical purposes and available in Europe from pharmacies at a reasonable cost. At the time of writing it is not yet readily available in the USA, but can be ordered by pharmacies. The side effects linked to Normast are negligible and it can be taken in addition to regular medication without fear of interactions or problems with tolerance. The most effective dose is 600mg daily.

As side effects commonly limit the use of many analgesics in fibromyalgia, especially for treating neuropathic pain, Normast appears to be a useful alternative. If you don't have neuropathic pain, this natural painkiller may not actually help you, but owing to its safety you can't cause yourself harm by trying it for a while. Any positive effects are evident within a few weeks.

4

Self-help measures for reducing pain

Pain is one of the body's chief survival mechanisms; it is the prompt that makes us act with urgency when an injury occurs. When pain arises without the trigger of an injury, however, and when it seems to be present for most of the time, all areas of life can be difficult to manage and it's common to feel thoroughly worn down. It doesn't help that fibromyalgia comes with a multitude of accompanying symptoms.

The main symptom is, of course, pain – persistent pain. If you don't have this, you don't have fibromyalgia. The pain is known to be more constant than in osteoarthritis and more intense than in conditions like rheumatoid arthritis and multiple sclerosis. It can be described as aching, burning, throbbing, searing or gnawing. Some people have even said that it's like a thousand jabbing needles. For many, the pain is widespread; for others, it is localized – focused on an area that's been overworked, such as the muscles, tendons and ligaments in a particular region. Or the pain can even veer between widespread and localized, usually depending upon what you have been doing.

Fibromyalgia pain can start out as localized, then gradually spread to further areas. For instance, it may begin in a person's shoulder or the base of their back, and over time extend throughout their body until eventually their whole body hurts. And, of course, the pain seems to interfere with every area of life – relationships, work, chores, interests, hobbies and recreational activities. Functional impairment also commonly occurs and many 'normal' movements such as bending, reaching, turning and even walking may become problematic. Having said that, the main reason that a small number of people with fibromyalgia use a wheelchair at times is more to combat the fatigue; or there may be another health issue such as hypermobility syndrome, a problem of joint laxity due to abnormal connective tissues.

Many onlookers find it difficult to understand that we may feel fine as we carry out an activity, but then often experience rising pain afterwards. For most people, the payback comes on fairly quickly; for some it doesn't arrive until the next day. This delay in the pain response can make it difficult for us to determine our triggering factors. On carefully looking back, though, we usually remember what we did that was out of our general routine.

Reasons for pain worsening

Because the pain of fibromyalgia is so easily exacerbated, it's important that we make efforts to understand what makes for added pain and what may trigger flare-ups. It's common for the following factors to aggravate fibromyalgia pain:

- *Overworking your body* – in fibromyalgia it is never wise to over-exert yourself, for example by lifting something too heavy or carrying out a repetitive action. We all have different tolerance levels and need to learn how much we can do before it gets too much. Listening to your body will usually tell you how much you can handle before there is an increase in pain. Remember that your tolerance levels are likely to keep changing. When you are feeling a little better, you may be able to carry out an activity you could not a few months earlier, so long as you proceed with care. On the other hand, there may be times when you are not up to tackling something you could previously have managed quite easily. In this case, you need time to strengthen your muscles before slowly getting back to where you were.
- *Holding out your arms or maintaining some kind of stretching action for too long* – in fibromyalgia, the muscles dislike being contracted for any length of time, and will start to complain. It is best to keep your arms relaxed and close to your sides as much as possible. If you need to reach out for something, try to assess whether your body can truly cope with the strain, or whether it would be wise to ask for help.
- *Emotional stress* – fibromyalgia can respond badly to emotional stress, such as that engendered by major events like a relationship break-up, the death of someone close, or your house being burgled, and so on. To temper your reactions to difficult situations and generally reduce your stress levels, try following a daily relaxation routine, such as those described on pages 92–4. You might benefit from listening to a relaxation CD. If you continue to be troubled by an issue in your life, why not have some counselling? You could perhaps ask your doctor for

a recommendation. Prescribed anti-stress medications can also help to get you over a crisis.

- *Certain weather conditions* – people with fibromyalgia often respond badly to cold damp weather, cold draughts and sudden climatic changes. It's common for symptoms to be much worse during the winter months than they are during summer, and for sudden changes in weather to trigger a worsening of pain or full flare-up. The best climate for fibromyalgia is warm and dry – that's why I relocated to the Canary Islands a few years ago. Hot humid climates are not usually great for us.

I must add that it's not always possible to pinpoint the exact cause of a pain exacerbation. To make matters worse, the pain can worsen for no apparent reason. That's fibromyalgia, I'm afraid.

Managing the pain

Avoiding your triggers is one of the chief aims in pain management. I realize that this is far easier said than done, especially where the weather and unforeseen emotional stresses are concerned. Keep yourself as warm and comfortable as possible and stay away from draughts. As for stresses – critical events such as a death in the family will always put you at risk of a flare-up, but smaller emotional stresses can be managed if you learn how to stay more relaxed in general (see pages 92–4 for information on relaxation).

If you suspect that another factor is aggravating your pain, try your best to identify it and then do something about it. For instance, you may have been told repeatedly that your posture is poor, in which case you would be well advised to start walking 'tall' and relaxed. Always choose the most supportive chair and sit fully on the seat with a small cushion behind you to create a gentle 'S' shape in your back. Finding out about the Alexander Technique might be a good option here too. Good posture is discussed in my book *Living with Fibromyalgia* (see Further reading at the back of this book).

You may believe that eating certain foods makes you feel worse temporarily, or brings on a flare-up. If this is the case, try hard to avoid that food. It's common in fibromyalgia to react badly to alcohol, too. A small sip of the stuff makes my muscles hypersensitive, after which they start to burn as if acid is searing through them. I'll sleep badly that night and wake up with a full-blown flare-up the next day. At the moment, though, I can manage to drink half a glass of white wine without repercussions, but any more than that and I wish that I had not bothered.

If you are still working full-time, I must congratulate you! You may feel, however, that the physical aspect of your job is exacerbating your pain, in which case is it possible to ask if you can be given a less physically demanding role; or maybe you should consider working part-time? Some jobs will always be difficult for people with fibromyalgia and you may need to look for lighter work. A job that is overly stressful can also have a negative effect on your health and there may be a need for a change here, too. A less important role in life may feel like a terrible come-down, but what good is having a high-ranking career when you are in more pain than you need be? I think that most of us would choose less pain and a decent family/social life over a great job that makes us feel ill and greatly limits other areas of our lives. If job satisfaction is of vital importance to you, there are usually alternative occupations that provide that, if you look hard enough for them.

Heat or cool?

We have long known that hot and cold therapy can success-fully ease pain. Often what works best is to use 'alternating treat-ment' – placing a bag of frozen peas, say, for five minutes on the painful area, swapping it for a warm gel pack (available from some pharmacies) for a further five minutes. After 20–30 minutes of this treatment, you can expect to feel better, and carrying it out once every two hours can be very helpful.

It's not always useful to apply heat only, especially if a hot, swollen joint is involved. With any suspicion of inflammation, cold application is far more effective – indeed, the application of heat can easily worsen inflammation. To see what works best for you, try different combinations of hot and cold.

Warm water exercise

Numerous studies have shown that warm water exercise is good for reducing pain, tender points, brain fog, anxiety and depression. In fact, it generally makes us feel better overall, for the warm water stops our muscles from tensing up and the buoyancy minimizes the pull of gravity, making our movements far less jarring. A thera-peutically heated pool should be set at around 32 degrees Celsius.

Action for flare-ups

Flare-ups always take us by surprise – and when I say flare-ups I mean the onset of fibromyalgia symptoms far more severe than our usual 'baseline' state. (Our baseline is how we normally are on a day-to-day basis, given that we have fibromyalgia.) When we overdo things in some way we are quite used to having an exacerbation in symptoms, but it is when that exacerbation will not 'rest off' during the next few hours that we can call it a flare-up. A true flare-up will last for one full day at the very least, and for several months in some cases.

There is always a reason – a trigger – for a flare-up, and it is important that you try to recognize it each time. You can then make an effort to avoid the circumstance in future. If the trigger is ongoing, such as a bout of insomnia or an episode of emotional stress, the flare-up may be prolonged unless you take positive action of some kind, such as getting medical help or embarking upon a course of counselling or hypnotherapy.

If you make no effort to calm the flare-up – for example, if you are continuing to look after your friend's baby when the job is really too difficult for you – the flare-up is liable to continue and lead to a rapid decline in your condition. In this instance, you would need to be honest and say that regretfully you really can't help your friend any longer as it's harming your health. Here, a true friend would probably express sorrow for imposing on you for so long and immediately look elsewhere for her babysitter.

As well as removing the cause of the flare-up, you can get it under control as quickly as possible by taking the following advice:

- At the outset, recognize when your pain levels are rising and take your painkillers before they increase further.
- Keep warm.
- Get plenty of rest on a comfortable but supportive surface, such as a bed with an orthopaedic mattress.
- Use pain-reliever rubs, such as Traumeel (available online), Ibuleve or Radian B. Or try mixing ginger oil, rose geranium and almond oil for a pain-relieving massage oil.
- Use a TENS machine.
- Take warm baths, using relaxing aromatherapy oils if they help. Adding Epsom salts to bathwater can also ease aches and pains, although this hasn't been researched much.

- Gently move your body every few minutes, even if you are lying in bed.
- Drink plenty of water.
- Take painkillers every four hours. If you use two types of painkillers, carefully alternate them. It is best to ask your doctor beforehand about this.
- Be positive! A positive frame of mind makes for a speedy recovery. Tell yourself: 'I'll get through this just as I have before'; 'I am more aware now of how to help myself'; 'I'll distract myself by listening to my music and audio books'; 'I won't feel sorry for myself – it doesn't help'.
- Explore the possible reasons for an increase in pain. Ask yourself questions such as: 'Did I overexert myself?'; 'Did I forget to pace myself?'; 'Should I have driven the car when I was already feeling fragile?'; 'Was I leaning forward too much?'; 'Should I have walked up all those steps?'
- Consider employing the help of a reflexologist, Reiki instructor, homeopath, acupuncturist, kinesiologist, chiropractor or osteopath.
- Fill your rest time with something that interests you, such as listening to talking books on CD or MP3 formats. Consider learning a language or something similar via 'listening' means. Watch your favourite DVDs, listen to the music you like, and so on. Try to place the things you need around you in case of a flare-up.
- Listen to a relaxation CD and regularly perform a relaxation routine.
- If you live alone, or look after children, have ready meals or frozen meals prepared earlier available to warm up. When (and if) you feel well enough to cook, it's a great idea to make extra meals and store them in the freezer for use during flare-ups.
- Inform people around you that you'll be out of action for a while.
- Once you start to feel better, be careful not to overdo things. Overdoing it too soon is the main reason for a flare-up persisting.
- If the flare-up won't seem to improve, no matter what you do, ask your doctor to visit.
- Decide how you can reduce the risk of future flare-ups. Do this by asking for help when you need it; by being clearer to others about what you can and can't do, and by lowering your expectations of yourself and others.
- Review the effectiveness of your current flare-up strategy. Are

your present medications adequate in a crisis? Can you do anything further to help you stay positive? Could you try a new type of complementary therapy? Is it time to visit your doctor again?

Pain and the emotions

Living with chronic pain has a huge impact on our lives, not least because it stirs strong feelings of loss. We may have lost our hoped-for future, we may have waved goodbye to our job, associated status and financial security, and we may have lost friends, perhaps people we felt close to but who have sadly proved to be fair-weather friends only. Fibromyalgia may have signified an end to light-hearted socializing and enjoyable nights out, at the cinema, restaurant or pub, or forced us to give up our particular hobbies and interests, perhaps the way we used to love slamming the ball around on the volleyball court. It hurts, too, that we are no longer able to interact with our children or grandchildren as we would wish, as it's difficult now to take them to the seaside, theme parks or on country walks.

Losing our hopes and dreams as well as the sense of our place in the world means that we can lose our sense of identity and our self-esteem sinks into our boots. It doesn't help that certain people can't seem to trust what we are telling them, and are perhaps critical of our efforts to get stronger. We can't help yearning for things to be as they once were – but they are clearly a million miles away, and that can be scary, to say the least.

Grieving for the things you have lost is normal in chronic pain. It's a natural emotion that most of us endure before we finally accept that things have changed for ever. It's important to remember, though, that your life has not necessarily changed for the worse – or if it seems that way at present, it can just as easily reverse when you start taking positive action. Yes, you have a chronic pain condition to manage, but with patience you can learn to incorporate its management into your new life. In time, pain management becomes second nature.

If you are still attempting to suppress negative feelings (such as anger, frustration and grief), try writing down your feelings; say them out loud several times, or even shout them at the top of your voice – perhaps when you are alone! This can be cathartic and helps you to move on.

How to move on

This section breaks down the chief requirements for moving forward with your life. If you are unable to follow them all, please don't worry. Taking just one or two on board will help you in your quest for improvement. You may be able to follow more of the advice at a later date, when you feel stronger.

Work with your doctor

It is essential that you are happy with the medical care you are receiving. If this is not the case, don't think twice about changing your doctor – perhaps one recommended by someone you trust. Always speak to your doctor respectfully and listen carefully to his or her comments. If you think that your doctor is failing to understand a particular aspect of your condition, be careful not to show irritation. Instead, using a calm, reasonable tone, repeat your problem in different words until you are satisfied that you are understood. If you have heard about a particular medication and would like to give it a try, mention this to your doctor very politely. For instance, you might say, 'I've been reading about so and so and it seems to be helping a lot of people. Do you think I might try it?' If your doctor seems reluctant and there is no obvious reason – for instance, it doesn't interact with your current medications and you don't have a risk factor for the medication, such as high blood pressure – you could say, 'If you don't mind, I'd really like to try it.'

It is very useful to have a reliable support network. As well as your doctor, this could include close family and friends, therapists, a support group and your rheumatologist, if you have one. A good support network can give you the strength to make positive changes.

Listen to your body

Perhaps the most important advice anyone can give you in fibromyalgia is to listen to your body. Allow it to tell you when you need to do the following:

* *Take a rest.* When you feel the first grips of increasing pain, take action and either sit or lie down. Some people can get away with resting comfortably in a chair for an hour before resuming an activity, others need to lie in bed for two to three hours before doing more. If you ignore the warning signs, you must expect an increase in pain. Ignoring the signs repeatedly can send you into a downward spiral in which you need more and more rest.

Your body may slowly grow weaker and be gripped by increasing amounts of pain.

- *Move around to loosen tight muscles.* If you have no choice but to spend a long time sitting – perhaps waiting at an appointment to see the doctor or dentist – keep getting up to circle your shoulders gently and swing your arms. You might also take yourself through a relaxation exercise, perhaps imagining yourself in a peaceful meadow by a gently trickling stream – and try hard not to worry. Staying as physically and mentally relaxed as possible will definitely help.
- *Eat and drink.* Eat and drink when your body tells you to, which should be about every three hours. Skipping a meal is not advisable in fibromyalgia, for if you fail to keep your glucose levels stable, you risk a huge dip in energy. Drink as much water as you can to keep your systems functioning as smoothly as possible, but drink fewer caffeine products (coffee, cocoa, cola drinks) and alcohol. Caffeine and alcohol cause an energy surge that is quickly followed by a slump into fatigue.
- *Indulge yourself.* When you are feeling anxious or stressed, do something that makes you feel relaxed and uplifted. This could be taking a long hot bath (perhaps with relaxing aromatherapy oils), having a massage, getting a new haircut, or having a manicure or pedicure or some other treatment that appeals to you. Or how about phoning your best friend to have a chat, buying yourself that new novel you fancied, watching your favourite film on DVD or listening to your favourite music.
- *Sleep.* If you are at home and start to feel sleepy, even if it is during the afternoon, escape to bed for a short nap. Go to bed at night as soon as you feel sleepy. Don't risk getting overtired as this will make sleep difficult to achieve later on.

Don't forget to do other things that are good for you, such as eating a healthy diet and taking plenty of exercise.

Interests and activities

If at all possible, try to replace the interests and activities that you can no longer do with interests and activities that you *are* able to do. Many people with chronic illness turn to more sedentary hobbies, which may be such things as playing computer games, card-making, sketching, making jewellery, song-writing, model-making, even playing a musical instrument. Occupying yourself with a hobby that you enjoy will give you a sense of achievement and help boost your self-esteem. Whatever interest you take up, though, it's important not to get so engrossed in it that you forget to pace yourself.

Many people with fibromyalgia even find that they can, at some point, go back to activities that they had been forced to abandon, so long as they employ pacing and avoid overexerting themselves.

Getting on with relatives

Sometimes it's tempting to keep our troubles to ourselves. We worry that opening up will scare off the people we care about or make them think that we're exaggerating or being plain dishonest. However, keeping everything inside means carrying a great load around – a load that is already over-heavy. It's therefore always advisable to tell family and friends how you are feeling – not every day, of course, but keep them in touch with your general position. If you are careful not to overburden them with your problems, they're likely to want to help or at least show that they understand.

Don't fight the pain

I found that when I stopped regarding fibromyalgia as my enemy, and when I ceased trying to fight it, it felt like a great pressure was no longer bearing down on me. I certainly didn't feel as if I was 'giving in' to the illness, for indeed I was not. I was accepting it as part and parcel of my life, as a small portion of what makes up the overall me.

The fibromyalgia part of us has very definite needs of its own, as has every other part of an individual, whatever that may be. This particular part is a rather demanding entity and we must allow it to have its say and we must look for ways to calm it down and make it feel better. In other words, pander to its whims and it should allow you to live an enjoyable life.

A new course in life

Fibromyalgia may dictate that you give up your job and look for a new course in life. There is nothing to say, however, that the new course cannot be just as rewarding, if not more so, than the old course was. I know plenty of people with fibromyalgia who have developed a hobby into a small business and are now having the time of their lives. I also know others who have chosen to retrain in a totally different field and love it so much, they wish they had taken the step years before. Counselling is a popular choice, I've noticed, for those whose self-esteem is fully restored. If counselling appeals to you, choose the type that doesn't cause you undue stress. Being a bereavement counsellor, for example, is not recommended for people with a chronic illness.

Before you look for your different course, take the time to accept that you have lost the future you had hoped for, that there is now a new part of yourself that is very demanding, then try to focus on forging a new way ahead. It's not sensible to sit back, do nothing, and simply expect that one day your doctor will offer a magic cure.

Your income

If you can claim disability benefits and so on, it's not important to look for a pastime that pays. It's far better to find something that most suits your personality and aptitude, makes you feel good about yourself, and is within your physical scope. We are all good at something – don't let low self-esteem stop you from recognizing your forte.

I'm sure you appreciate that having money isn't the be-all and end-all in life. So long as there is sufficient to live on, sufficient to enjoy yourself with, within reason, that really should be enough. If your finances are very tight and there is nothing at all left over for unexpected mishaps or a little enjoyment, don't hesitate to request advice from your local social services.

Lifestyle principles

For the best outcome of all, healthwise, you would be well advised to follow certain lifestyle principles. It's rare for lasting improvement to come about in fibromyalgia without a concerted effort to observe these principles.

The lifestyle principles that are vital to improvement include the following:

- Adopt a daily gentle exercise routine, such as that described in my book *Living with Fibromyalgia* and other exercise books.
- Use pacing. Alternate rest periods with gentle activity throughout the day so you don't overtax yourself.
- Listen to your body. Stop what you are doing as soon as you experience rising discomfort.
- Be proactive in your treatment. Read all you can about fibromyalgia and what treatments and therapies are likely to help, then put what you have read into action. Try to be clear-minded about what you need to do.

- Eat a healthy balanced diet. See Chapter 6 for diet information, or read my book *The Fibromyalgia Healing Diet* for details of the best food choices for people with fibromyalgia.
- Keep warm and stay out of draughts. Take plenty of warm baths, if they help.
- Find things to do that give you a sense of achievement.
- Don't be afraid to discuss your problems with others.
- Work with your doctor. If you don't find your doctor helpful, find someone else.
- Keep a diary to help identify your triggers for flare-ups. Record details of your everyday life, diet, sleep, activity levels, and if you are stressed by anything at the time. You should see a pattern emerging in which your triggers are revealed. Now try to adapt your lifestyle in a way that reduces your triggers.
- Keep your stress levels as low as possible. Try to avoid over-reacting to stressful situations and practise a daily relaxation routine. In your diary, note the persons, places, activities and situations that make you feel stressed. If you can avoid a particular stressor, do. If not, do whatever it takes to help you cope better. For example, if certain friends make you feel stressed, try to limit your interactions with them. If you find driving stressful, get lifts with friends or neighbours, or take the bus or a taxi. If you find going to the supermarket stressful, ask someone to accompany you, or try online shopping.

I realize that it's not always possible to follow these lifestyle principles to the letter, every day. Perhaps you're simply not well enough to exercise, or cook a healthy meal, in which case it's acceptable to give yourself time off. However, don't forget to recommence your exercise routine as soon as you can, at a slightly less 'advanced' stage, and slowly build up to where you were. Where food is concerned, it's always best to plan ahead in fibromyalgia, making extra meals when you are up to it to store in the freezer. Alternatively, ask a family member or close friend to help by preparing a stock of healthy meals for you; or even keep a supply of healthy-option microwave meals in the freezer for when all else fails. If you live alone and are not up to cooking or looking after a home, ask your local social services for urgent help.

If you are able to build all the above principles into your daily life and stick to them most of the time, you should find that your pain levels and flare-ups gradually decrease.

5

Help for other symptoms

Because so many symptoms are part and parcel of fibromyalgia – symptoms that on the face of it are unrelated – it's no wonder that some of us fear we are going mad, or worry about being seen as hypochondriacs. It takes time to absorb the fact that the symptoms are all interconnected somehow, and it can take even longer for family and friends to reach that conclusion. Explaining to others that fibromyalgia is a multi-system, whole-body disorder, causing a number of different kinds of problems, isn't at all easy, but it is definitely worth trying. You could also show any doubters one or two of the many books on the subject, pointing out the symptoms section in particular.

Don't let people who treat you like a hypochondriac cause you grief and upset. If you know that you've tried your best to make them understand but they simply won't, it's advisable to slowly drop them from your life. If that isn't possible, grit your teeth and bear it. It's they who have the problem, not you – and having poor empathy in general doesn't make for a happy life.

Fatigue

Fatigue is almost universal in fibromyalgia. It has been described as an overwhelming heaviness of the arms and legs, as if they are full of concrete. Some of us only notice the tiredness after perhaps traipsing around the shops for a couple of hours, whereas others feel constantly drained, and for no reason other than it is part of our fibromyalgia. We can even feel too fatigued to communicate properly, which obviously can affect our relationships.

Waking up exhausted, and not improving during the day, can be just as difficult emotionally as constantly being in pain. Indeed, some unfortunate people are as troubled by fatigue as they are by pain. A person who wakes up exhausted, however, will normally 'pick up' a little as the day goes on, whereas pain will normally worsen.

As mentioned earlier, chronic fatigue syndrome (CFS) is a similar condition to fibromyalgia. However, the pain is more dominant in fibromyalgia and the fatigue is more dominant in CFS. If you have been diagnosed with fibromyalgia yet your fatigue is excessive and often incapacitating, a diagnosis of CFS may also be given. The treatments for both conditions are very similar. Pacing is important, as is gentle exercise, a healthy diet and the appropriate medications (your doctor will give guidance regarding medications). Note that in the UK, CFS is often referred to as myalgic encephalomyelitis (ME).

In fibromyalgia, the following factors are usually associated with fatigue:

- *Non-restorative sleep* – in deep sleep, the growth hormones prolactin and testosterone rise appreciably, facilitating tissue repair and regeneration. Healthy people have these hormones in good supply, but people with fibromyalgia have a significant shortfall due to our inability to achieve deep sleep.
- *Deconditioned muscles* – normal muscles make an energy molecule called adenosine triphosphate (ATP), which enables them to perform all their functions with ease. In fibromyalgia, our out-of-condition muscles can stop manufacturing this fuel, which contributes to chronic fatigue.
- *Poor oxygen use* – in fibromyalgia the muscles fail to use energy as efficiently as normal muscles. This may be due to dysfunction of the tiny compounds that use oxygen to manufacture ATP.
- *Expressing pain* – when we are hurting all the time, our bodies use up energy faster than normal and have less stored energy. Also, our bodies naturally monitor and record our pain levels, which uses a lot of energy.
- *Depression* – the depression arising in fibromyalgia may cause extreme mental fatigue.

Assuming your fatigue is associated with your fibromyalgia and not linked with another health problem, it can be treated. Fatigue can be caused by anaemia, sleep disorders and an overactive thyroid, and these conditions require different treatment approaches.

If your fatigue is severe, your doctor may wish to take a sample of your blood to measure your blood count, and check for thyroid problems, growth hormone deficiency, a shortfall in magnesium and so on. If a problem is found, your doctor will take the appropriate steps.

Medications and supplements for fatigue

Many people with chronic fatigue find the following medications useful – although others gain no benefit at all. If you are not aware of improvement within three months of taking a medication or supplement, it's best to stop taking it.

- *Serotonin-enhancing medications* – the selective serotonin re-uptake inhibitors (SSRIs), such as Prozac (fluoxetine), Paxil (paroxetine), Serzone (nefazodone hydrochloride) and Zoloft (sertraline), can boost serotonin levels and so improve fatigue.
- *Magnesium and malic acid* – perhaps the most successful energy-boosting supplement is a magnesium and malic acid combination. It works by increasing the levels of energy formed in the muscle. Magnesium and malic acid with added colostrum is even better.
- *'B complex' vitamins* – the B complex vitamins are often very useful for improving pain, fatigue and stress. B12 may offer the best help. When taken in tablet form, B12 is sometimes not well absorbed into the blood, and it may now be administered by injection. Ask your doctor about this. B12 can also be taken in the form of a sublingual (suckable) tablet, and apparently a one-month course can make all the difference to fatigue and 'brain fog', especially if you are over 50 or don't eat much meat.
- *5-HTP* – a natural building block of serotonin, 5-HTP can help to improve sleep, stabilize mood and decrease pain. See page 100 for more information.

If depression is the root cause of a good deal of your fatigue, your doctor may prescribe an antidepressant medication. Improving depression usually improves fatigue.

Morning stiffness

Although the stiffness in fibromyalgia comes mainly from the areas where muscles and tendons attach to the joints, it's common to feel stiff all over. The stiffness is particularly pronounced after a prolonged period of immobility, such as after a month-long flare-up or if you have been wheelchair-bound for weeks or even months.

We may feel very stiff when we wake in a morning but normally improve as the day goes on. Some people are very stiff after sitting down for just 15 minutes, whereas others hardly experience stiffness at all.

Sleep problems

Most people with fibromyalgia have difficulty sleeping at night. Some have trouble getting off to sleep, some wake frequently during the night, and some wake too early and can't drop off again. Researchers looking at brainwave patterns during sleep in people with fibromyalgia found that most of us have a sleep disorder called the 'alpha-EEG anomaly' in which our stage 4 sleep – the deep level – is constantly interrupted by bursts of brain activity similar to that of being awake. This is one reason why we often wake feeling tired.

During stage 4 sleep as experienced by healthy people, levels of prolactin and testosterone – the growth hormones – rise significantly, facilitating tissue repair and boosting energy stores. Some repair work goes on in our inefficient fibromyalgia sleep, but it is invariably incomplete, as is the production of energy. As a result, we are likely to have growth hormones in short supply. However, they can be induced, to some extent, by changing to a high-protein diet, taking mineral supplements before bedtime and using relaxation techniques. If you have not already been prescribed tricyclic antidepressant medication (tricyclics can help to improve pain, sleep problems and low mood), it might be an idea to discuss the matter with your doctor. A short course of antidepressants can encourage your body into a better sleep rhythm.

The following tips can help you to sleep longer and more deeply:

- Take fewer daytime naps, and when you do, sleep for a shorter duration – no longer than half an hour. All naps, even those that are not energizing, can prevent you from feeling sleepy at bedtime.
- Hang heavy curtains to make the bedroom as dark as possible.
- Before trying to sleep, unwind by listening to music or a relaxation CD, reading, or watching an unexciting programme on TV.
- Have a warm drink.
- Shortly before bedtime, take a hot bath (preferably using relaxing aromatherapy oils).
- Go to bed when you feel sleepy, so long as it is not before 9.30 p.m.

- Ensure that your bed and bedroom are comfortably warm, but not overheated.
- Wear a sleep mask to cut out any light; this may help you to sleep soundly for longer.
- Use earplugs to eliminate distracting noises.
- Make yourself comfortable in bed, breathing slowly and evenly into your diaphragm. Clear your mind and allow your thoughts to drift. Don't hold on to any one thought, but let them pass unchecked.
- Set your alarm for the same time every morning.

Try to avoid:

- drinking caffeine after 6 p.m.;
- drinking alcohol before bedtime;
- eating, drinking or reading in bed;
- engaging in animated conversation (or arguments) before bedtime;
- sitting up to watch television for long periods in the evening.

Sitting to watch television for several hours during the daytime and evening not only causes stiffness and muscle pain, it also interferes with sleep. This is because television provokes numerous emotional responses in rapid succession, quickening the heart rate and releasing the 'on-alert' chemicals (such as adrenaline and cortisol) for no useful purpose. When these chemicals are produced naturally, we deal with the situation and our blood flow is returned to normal. But when chemicals are induced second-hand, as in watching television, they remain in the bloodstream. As a result, tension lingers, muscle pain increases and sleep is very difficult.

Sleep apnoea

Some people with fibromyalgia have a condition called sleep apnoea. This means that breathing during sleep is irregular, and you may even stop breathing for a short period. Fortunately, the body's natural defence mechanisms soon trigger the breathing reflex, and you start breathing again, without any harm being done.

Abnormal breathing prevents our batteries from being recharged and can contribute to tiredness and fatigue. Fortunately, it is possible to reduce sleep apnoea by following the general advice for improving fatigue and sleep.

How to encourage better sleep

Here are a few more tips for improving sleep:

- Pace yourself carefully throughout the day.
- Learn to say 'no', so you don't push yourself unnecessarily.
- Do something you enjoy every day, so long as it's within your physical scope.
- If possible, take a daily stroll – it doesn't have to be a long one. A short walk is better than no walk at all.
- If you go to work in a morning, get up 15 minutes earlier than usual so that you are not tempted to rush around.
- Eat a low-calorie, high-fibre breakfast such as grapefruit followed by porridge oats, or breakfast cereal followed by wholemeal toast. Avoid sugary cereals.
- Drink natural fruit juice at breakfast – not juices with added sugar or sweeteners. Alternatively, drink a glass of warm boiled water with freshly squeezed lemon juice.
- Stick to regular meal times and don't skip meals.
- Exercise in the morning. Avoid exercising in the six hours before bedtime.

Sleep medications

Over-the-counter sleep medications such as melatonin, valerian root, passion flower, kava kava and a 5-HTP and vitamin D3 combination (see below) can increase the duration of sleep. However, they cannot lengthen deep sleep, which is essential for tissue repair and energy production. You may, then, be prescribed a tricyclic antidepressant to encourage deep sleep. If you have used tricyclics previously but they don't work or are no longer effective, the dosage may require adjusting or you may need to try another type.

As some sleep medications – namely muscle relaxants – are habit-forming and become less effective over time, you can get the best out of them by rotating them with any other sleep medications you have. Try to use muscle relaxants on a short-term basis only, to urge you into a better sleep pattern.

Vitamin D3 (cholecalciferol)

It's possible to take a simple laboratory test to find out whether you are deficient in vitamin D3 – a hormone that is integral to the sleep process. If you are deficient, the vitamin is best taken in liquid form, placed by a dropper on to your tongue, before going to bed – 4,000IU, taken in two 2,000IU drops, seems to work best. If you are interested in this option, speak to your doctor.

As very high levels of vitamin D can cause toxicity problems, be careful to stay within the recommended limits. Vitamin D supplementation combined with a lot of sunshine, however – which makes vitamin D naturally in the body – would not be sufficient to cause problems.

5-HTP (5-hydroxytryptophan)

When vitamin D3 is taken in combination with a chemical called 5-HTP – which raises levels of serotonin, the sleep-inducing chemical – sleep patterns can revert to normal within a few days. It is recommended that 100–200mg of 5-HTP is taken daily with vitamin D3 until laboratory tests show that there is no longer a deficiency.

If you are suffering from depression as well as sleeplessness, you can take a 100mg dosage of 5-HTP three or four times daily without the need for laboratory tests beforehand. Depression often responds well to a return to normal sleeping, adrenal gland support (which 5-HTP offers), and vitamin and mineral therapy (see Chapter 6).

Daytime rest

When you need to rest during the day, it may be tempting to slump in front of the television for a couple of hours. This is fine for someone whose muscles don't tire easily and can cope with being stretched or scrunched for this length of time, but it is often counter-productive in fibromyalgia, and can make you feel just as weary and sore as beforehand. However, lying down on a comfortable and supportive surface can make a great difference to how quickly you can 'rest off' discomfort or an increase in pain.

Resting with your eyes open while lying down is a great way to relax and unwind (see 'Awareness meditation', pages 92–3).

Headaches and migraine

Up to 70 per cent of people with fibromyalgia have recurrent headaches, and they can be difficult to cope with. Headaches and migraines are caused by the constriction and dilation of the tiny capillaries bringing blood to the brain, and they can be triggered by anxiety, emotional stress, flickering lights and sensitivity to foods such as red wine, strong cheese, chocolate, caffeinated coffee and tea, alcohol and cured meats. Migraines are more severe than the 'tight elastic band' sensation of a tension headache, and are characterized by one-sided intense throbbing and sensitivity to light and sound. There may also be alterations in vision, nausea and sometimes vomiting.

As headaches gradually slow the digestion, it becomes increasingly difficult for the body to absorb treatments taken by mouth. Therefore, it is important to tackle a headache when you first notice it coming on.

You may gain sufficient relief from over-the-counter drugs such as aspirin, paracetamol or ibuprofen. If not, you could try taking Imigran Recovery – this contains sumatriptan, a 'triptan drug' which reduces the vascular inflammation associated with migraine. Imigran Recovery is available over the counter from pharmacies, usually on completion of a questionnaire to assess your suitability. Naratriptan, a similar triptan sulfa drug, is available only on prescription. It is best to take your chosen medication with a cup of coffee or glass of cola, as caffeine boosts the effectiveness of this type of painkiller and helps to reduce swollen blood vessels. Obviously, if caffeine is a migraine or headache trigger for you, it should be avoided.

If the attack is severe, you will need to rest in a darkened room, perhaps wearing an eye mask, until you feel much better. Some people find that a hot or cold compress on the site of the pain is very helpful. In my case, a drop of lavender oil regularly massaged into the painful area can work wonders. You should find, though, as I have, that your headaches or migraines reduce significantly as your general condition improves.

Irritable bowel syndrome (IBS)

IBS is characterized by frequent abdominal cramps and gas (wind), with bloating and pain. There are often alternating bouts of diarrhoea and constipation, but some people have just diarrhoea or just constipation. Although no damage is caused to the bowel, the symptoms are often distressing.

IBS is found in approximately 15 per cent of the general population, but in up to 70 per cent of the fibromyalgia population, which indicates, therefore, a clear link between the two conditions. In both fibromyalgia and IBS there is an altered pain response, with initial research suggesting that the nerves controlling the bowel and bladder (see pages 58–9 for information on irritable bladder) are linked to the nerves of the brain and central nervous system, from which pain signals arise. Researchers are very interested in why the two conditions appear to be linked.

Most of the symptoms in fibromyalgia come from dysfunctions in the muscles under voluntary control, but in IBS it is the so-called 'smooth muscles' under involuntary control that create the problem. Tests can be carried out to check for specific problems, but as your doctor may be used to their being returned marked 'normal', he or she may not bother. If you have severe IBS, your doctor may refer you to a colorectal specialist or proctologist.

Peppermint oil acts as a muscle relaxant, particularly in the digestive tract, and it can be used to great effect for the treatment of IBS. Take one or two enteric-coated peppermint capsules two or three times a day between meals. Each capsule should contain 0.2ml of oil. Many people drink peppermint tea every day as it offers a soothing option to capsules or tinctures.

Another natural option for IBS is to take flaxseed (linseed), which contains insoluble fibre and oil.

Yeast infection

IBS symptoms are often triggered by an adverse reaction to certain foods. The chief culprits include caffeine, chocolate, fatty foods, alcohol and fizzy drinks. People with intestinal candida – a yeast-like parasitic fungus that can cause thrush in women – tend to have more of a problem with IBS, which is made worse if they eat a lot of yeast products. These products include cheese, mushrooms, white bread, cakes, dried fruit, wine, beer, cider, vinegar, Bovril, Marmite, pickles, ketchup, salad dressing and products containing MSG (monosodium glutamate, a food additive).

Yeasts are a group of microscopic fungi, which may be present in our diet deliberately, as in baking and fermentation, or accidentally, as in over-ripe fruit and food that is past its best or its 'eat by' date. If you have a candida (chronic yeast) infection you would be advised to remove sugar from your diet, as sugar encourages the growth of yeast. And since IBS is exacerbated by yeast itself, all yeast products should also be removed.

Foods and treatments to improve IBS

Foods containing fibre can improve IBS – whole-grain breads, cereal, fresh fruits, beans and vegetables. The following treatments can also help to ease IBS:

- fibre supplements, to boost your fibre intake
- laxatives, to treat constipation
- antispasmodics, to decrease stomach cramps
- antidepressants, to decrease stomach cramps when antispasmodics alone don't work.

You may wish to ask your doctor or pharmacist to suggest something for your particular case.

Eating large meals will only worsen IBS, so you can improve the situation by reducing the size of your helpings. It is best to eat four or five small meals a day, with healthy IBS-friendly snacks in between.

Irritable bladder

It's common for women with fibromyalgia to have an irritable bladder as well as IBS. Indeed, they are 'sister' conditions. There are three types of bladder problem, as discussed below.

Urinary frequency

Many women with fibromyalgia and IBS have urinary frequency and abdominal bloating, the main symptoms of irritable bladder. They need to visit the toilet many times a day. It's not unusual for some to need to urinate every 20–30 minutes, which is time-consuming, frustrating and intrudes too much on daily life. Sleep can be severely disrupted by the sensations of a full bladder.

The signs of urinary frequency are:

- having a frequent urge to pass urine;
- having difficulty 'holding' urine;
- waking to pass urine more than once in the night;
- pain on urination.

Urinary urgency

Urinary urgency – the urgent need to pass urine – is also common in fibromyalgia. The desire to urinate can take you by surprise at times, making a visit to the toilet urgent. Some people become fearful of leaving home in case the urge takes them when no toilet is nearby.

The signs of urinary urgency include:

- having to pass urine frequently;
- sudden urges to pass urine immediately;

- pelvic pain or discomfort;
- times when you don't quite reach the toilet and an accident occurs;
- possible episodes of incontinence during the night, when you don't wake up in time.

Urinary incontinence

Urinary incontinence is particularly common in women, though few like to discuss it. The term describes the inability to control bladder function, making life embarrassing and frustrating. Many people link incontinence with ageing, but it's not always the case. Incontinence isn't common in fibromyalgia, but a small number are affected. Its cause is uncertain, but it may arise from weakened bladder muscles or even fatigue.

Treatment

If you have bladder problems, your doctor may wish to see a laboratory culture of your urine to rule out the presence of a urinary infection. In men, prostate secretions may be cultured to look for problems in the prostate gland. If infection or prostate problems are found, you will be offered the appropriate treatment.

There are several prescription medications aimed at improving bladder function, for example tricyclic antidepressants, and a drug called Detrusitol (tolterodine tartrate) which can strengthen bladder muscles. Your doctor should be able to prescribe the most appropriate drug. Some patients may be offered electrical stimulation to help retrain their bladder muscles, whereas others may require a surgical procedure to increase their bladder capacity.

It is also possible to regain bladder control by means of biofeedback sessions at a local hospital's outpatient department. Bladder control biofeedback teaches you to use regular pelvic floor exercises (known as Kegel exercises) to strengthen your bladder muscles, and it helps you to pass urine only at specific times of the day. The aim is to reduce the number of times you need to dash to the toilet.

Cognitive problems – 'fibro fog'

It's normal for someone with fibromyalgia to have problems with thinking. Indeed, we often mix up our words, find it difficult to concentrate and have short-term memory loss, absentmindedness, confusion and general mental fatigue – all of which are known as 'fibro fog'. Many of us fear that we are developing dementia or that our brain is being irrevocably damaged. Fortunately, neither is the case, for when we are not being 'ditzy' we are still able to absorb information and display normal memory and powers of thinking.

Modern scanning techniques have shown restricted blood flow in the parts of the brain controlling memory and concentration, which may be part of the problem. Also, the neurotransmitter problems in fibromyalgia can hamper clear thinking. It certainly doesn't help that we are chronically short of restorative sleep, constantly fatigued and feeling the effects of long-term pain.

Forgetfulness can be overcome, to some extent, by using a series of memory prompt techniques, such as always writing things down and keeping an appointments diary. Other cognitive problems can be improved by certain medications – speak to your doctor about these. You may also wish to try the herbal supplement ginkgo biloba, which boosts blood flow to the brain.

Anxiety

The endless barrage of fibromyalgia symptoms would create anxiety in anyone. It's not only that, either, for the autonomic nervous system doesn't function correctly in fibromyalgia, and that compounds the problem.

Chronically anxious people are edgy and oversensitive. They get upset more easily than usual and find it difficult to sleep. As a result, relaxation can be difficult to achieve – yet knowing how to relax is an important part of managing day-to-day life when you have a chronic condition. Moreover, relaxed muscles use far less energy than tense ones, and improved breathing leads to better circulation and oxygenation, which in turn helps the muscles and connective tissues. A calm, relaxed mind can also greatly aid concentration and short-term memory.

Chronic anxiety shows itself in a number of possible symptoms:

- excessive worrying
- sleep problems
- mood changes and irritability
- tremors and twitching
- increased muscle tension and therefore pain
- headache
- sweating and hot flushes

- light-headedness
- shortness of breath.

In order to cope with anxiety effectively, it's best to limit or cut out certain stimulants, particularly caffeine, alcohol and tobacco. Stimulants are known to exacerbate anxiety.

If you are unable to relieve your anxiety yourself, it's important that you visit your doctor. You are likely to be offered a course of benzodiazepines or antidepressants (either tricyclic or an SSRI). It may also be recommended that you have some counselling.

Panic attacks

A panic attack is acute hyperventilation, or 'over-breathing', in response to an anticipated threat. Sometimes the perceived threat is obvious, but in chronic anxiety there is often no obvious reason for the onset of panicky feelings.

Panic attacks are preceded by intensifying anxiety. The individual starts breathing faster in troubled apprehension, exhaling far more carbon dioxide than is normal. The result is light-headedness, palpitations and the sensation that the chest is tightening, accompanied by feelings of inadequacy, fear, and maybe impending doom.

An immediate remedy is the good old paper bag. Place the bag over your nose and mouth and try to breathe more slowly. Breathing into the bag will ensure that most of the exhaled carbon dioxide is returned to your lungs. Daily deep breathing exercises – where breathing is slowed down and on inhalation the abdomen (not the ribcage) is allowed to rise – are very useful training.

It's important that you seek the help of your doctor if you suffer from panic attacks. Again, you are likely to be prescribed a course of antidepressants or benzodiazepines, and if past or present life events are troubling you, you may be referred to a counsellor.

Panic attacks are fairly common in anxiety conditions.

Depression

It's common to feel 'low' for a while every now and again, but that's not depression. True depression makes you feel sad all the time, for many months or even longer. It also means a loss of self-esteem, feelings of hopelessness and a lack of interest in the things you used to enjoy.

Depression is a disabling condition that affects life on all levels – your interactions with family, ability to work, social life, eating and sleeping habits and general health. In addition, it's common to be preoccupied with inappropriate guilt or regret and self-loathing, and to feel constantly fatigued, suffer headaches and swing between agitation and lethargy.

Life events can sometimes trigger depression, especially if you are predisposed to it anyway. Common triggers are bereavement, divorce, having a baby or being bullied. It's also possible to develop depression for no apparent reason, in which case hormonal dysfunction is probably the root cause. The hormone serotonin is present at an abnormally low level in both depression and fibromyalgia, and this links the two conditions. Note that even though true depression is found in around 50 per cent of people with fibromyalgia, it doesn't automatically follow that if you have fibromyalgia you have, or are going to get, depression.

In short, the symptoms of depression include:

- being tearful, with persistent sadness and feelings of hopelessness;
- feeling lethargic and sapped of energy;
- low self-esteem and feelings of worthlessness;
- being unable to enjoy things that were once pleasurable;
- slow-motion thinking and behaviour;
- irritability and intolerance of others;
- headaches and unexplained aches and pains;
- constant anxiety;
- difficulty sleeping or sleeping too much;
- diminished sex drive or erectile dysfunction in men;
- either a loss of appetite or a ravenous appetite;
- thoughts of suicide and even suicide attempts.

If you think you are depressed but have not yet seen your doctor, please do so straight away. The sooner you get help the sooner you should find yourself on the road to recovery.

Treatment usually involves a combination of medication and a 'talking' therapy. Medications may include tricyclic antidepressants and SSRIs. Some people try more natural therapies such as SAMe (see page 99) or 5-HTP (see pages 100–1), but in truth these are only useful for mild depression. For the talking therapy, you may be referred to a psychologist at your local hospital, where, among other things, you will be taught relaxation and some very useful techniques for overcoming certain problems.

You can help yourself by getting plenty of exercise, eating healthily, cutting down on alcohol and perhaps joining a support group for people with depression.

Hypersensitivity

In fibromyalgia, our nervous systems have become hypersensitive. Therefore, many everyday things create an adverse reaction.

People with fibromyalgia can have the following sensitivity problems:

- *It's common to react adversely to environmental chemicals.* These include pesticides, artificial fertilizers, petro-chemical fumes, glue, varnish, aerosol sprays, and some air fresheners, household cleaners, paints and perfumes. Some fibromyalgia symptoms are greatly exacerbated by chemical exposure.
- *Chemical and other food additives* can cause a problem. The most common culprits are the chemical additives and preservatives present in processed foods – that is, foods that have been altered from their natural state for convenience and a longer shelf-life. Processing methods include canning, spray-drying, freeze-drying, refrigeration, dehydration and the introduction of artificial sweeteners, colouring agents and preservatives. Also, processed foods are often made with trans-fats, saturated fats and copious amounts of sodium and sugar, which are detrimental to health. It is best to consume processed foods very sparingly. Monosodium glutamate (MSG) is a particular worry, yet this is added to thousands of food items every day.
- *Some everyday foods can trigger a physical reaction,* anything from a light headache and indigestion to migraine, diarrhoea and fierce stomach cramps. It's even possible to suffer the life-threatening allergic reaction known as anaphylactic shock, a condition in which the airway rapidly constricts and breathing is difficult. In anaphylaxis, an injection of adrenaline is required as a matter of urgency to calm the reaction. Many people with fibromyalgia have an adverse reaction of some kind after consuming a certain food or drink. The most problematic foods are gluten, nuts, shellfish, caffeine and dairy products. And if eating yeast-containing foods causes you to experience stomach cramps, bloating and so on, eliminate them from your diet for a while. As yeast infections are aggravated by sugar, it's also best to cut down on sugary foods.

- *You may be allergic to pollen* from grass, flowers and trees – this is hay fever. It can cause a streaming nose and eyes, sneezing, headache, congestion, sore throat and many other unpleasant symptoms, which normally last for several weeks during the spring and summer when there is a lot of pollen in the air.
- *Certain medications* can also cause problems. We don't always tolerate prescribed medications and can experience troublesome side effects. The most likely offenders are aspirin and SSRIs, penicillin, streptomycin, insulin and vaccinations, particularly against flu and measles. Often the side effects are worse than the problem for which we initially took the medication or injection! If side effects are at all bothersome, it's important to inform your doctor. There is likely to be a less troublesome alternative. Our children should always have the measles vaccination, though, as a wide resurgence of measles would be a terrific health risk.
- *Sensitivity to the weather* – cold weather, cold and damp weather, and occasionally hot and humid weather can trigger flare-ups. Most of us cope best in a warm, dry climate.
- *Loud noises* can be unbearable, causing tinnitus, headache and irritability.
- *Bright light* can give rise to headache, eye strain and visual disturbances.
- *Dust* can cause sneezing and congestion in some people.

Chemical sensitivities

Chemical sensitivity is present in about 50 per cent of fibromyalgia cases. It can give rise to fatigue, headaches, nausea, short-term memory loss, mood changes, and numbness and tingling in the fingers and toes. It is even believed to restrict blood flow to and through the parts of the brain dealing with pain regulation, memory and concentration. Interestingly, apart from a few exceptions, it is no coincidence that in countries with little industrial power, and where fresh food is eaten straight from the land, there is generally a marked low allergy situation.

Sensitization to chronic chemical exposure is now well documented. It has been known for mechanics to become sensitized to petrol fumes, painters to paint, printers to ink, and so on. Maybe we should all take a closer look at our immediate environments. Eliminating, or at least reducing, specific trigger factors could greatly improve fibromyalgia. Triggers are not always easy to spot, however. Many medical professionals maintain that a healthy diet, rest, relaxation and plenty of exercise can help increase the body's tolerance of chemicals.

People with fibromyalgia often have a keen sense of smell, which means that they can be more affected by smells than others.

Natural cleaning products

- Half a lemon can be used to clean, degrease, bleach and disinfect. Use to clean the bath, toilet and washbasin, and to shine the taps.
- White vinegar can be used to clean, degrease, disinfect and deodorize. Use to clean tiles, worktops and windows, afterwards buffing windows with crumpled newspaper.
- White vinegar, mixed with several drops of your favourite essential oil, can be poured into a spray bottle and used as a natural air freshener.
- Olive oil, mixed with lemon juice, is a natural alternative for commercial furniture polish. Pour into a spray bottle.
- Bicarbonate of soda, mixed with water, helps to dissolve dirt and grease, neutralize smells and remove carpet stains.

Dizziness

Another common symptom in fibromyalgia is chronic dizziness. The majority of the general population will have experienced dizziness at some point in their lives, and know it as a momentary sensation of light-headedness, where the world seems to spin and they need to either grab on to something or sit down for fear of falling. The spell is soon over for most people, though, and they can get back to what they were doing. When dizzy spells are frequent and prolonged (in fibromyalgia, they can last from a few seconds to several days), life can become difficult. In my case, putting my head down can make everything spin for a few seconds; the problem lasts for a few months at a time before mysteriously correcting itself. Of course, I try hard to avoid this particular movement, but that's not easy, especially in the shower, and I'm only grateful for the grab rail on the shower wall.

In normal dizziness, problems arise from mixed messages received by our brain from our 'equilibrium system'. This system is based in our ears, eyes, skin and muscles, all of which send messages to our brains to keep us steady, balanced and headed in the right direction. However, our equilibrium system is easily confused by certain messages. For instance, bouncing on a trampoline with our eyes fixed on one spot prevents our brains from knowing where exactly we are in space. The result can be dizziness and perhaps nausea.

In fibromyalgia the problem is thought to be linked to the body's inability to circulate blood efficiently. To be more specific, we often have 'neurally mediated hypotension', which means that our bodies don't find it easy to regulate our blood pressure. When I bow my head, the blood stops rising to my brain and the result is dizziness. Other people can feel dizzy on rising from a chair or bed, for the blood suddenly rushes to their lower extremities. The heart should respond to sudden posture changes by pumping more blood around the body and up into the brain, but this doesn't always happen in fibromyalgia – hence the dizziness and fainting or near-fainting, where your vision becomes blurred or you experience a vision 'blackout' or other symptoms. The most common symptoms associated with dizziness include the following:

- blurred vision or a vision 'blackout'
- sweating or cold chills
- fainting or near-fainting
- headache
- tinnitus or other hearing problems.

Unfortunately, there is little the medical profession can do for fibromyalgia-related dizziness. Still, if you are experiencing this symptom, see your doctor about it as the cause may be something you hadn't considered. For instance, chronic hypotension – long-term low blood pressure – can cause dizziness. (Hypotension is the opposite of hypertension, which is long-term high blood pressure, while neurally mediated hypotension is sudden drops in blood pressure due to postural changes.) Chronic hypotension usually responds well to appropriate medication.

Other causes of dizziness can arise from anywhere in the equilibruim system, the ears being a common culprit. If your doctor finds a problem anywhere in this system, you will be offered helpful medication, such as anti-emetic drugs.

If there is no obvious cause for the dizziness, your doctor will put it down to your fibromyalgia. It then becomes just another of the many symptoms we have to manage. If the dizziness is severe, however, treatment is available to counter the problem.

Chest pains

Many people with fibromyalgia experience pains in their chest and ribcage – known as costochondritis. In fact, it is often the first symptom of fibromyalgia. Costochondritis can seem to mimic heart attack pain, but it is not usually a sign of heart problems.

Costochrondritis is caused by inflammation of the cartilage that attaches the ribs to the breast bone (sternum), and sometimes all the seven junction points can be affected. The inflammation gives rise to sharp pains inside the chest wall, and there is tenderness or pain when the area is pressed. Women between the ages of 20 and 40 are most likely to develop this condition, especially those with larger breasts. The pain will normally wax and wane, perhaps lasting for several weeks or months before disappearing for a spell.

Possible symptoms of fibromyalgia-related costochondritis are as follows:

- sharp pains in the front of the chest
- a burning pain in the ribs
- ribs that are sore when touched
- pain on one side of the chest
- pain that increases on activity, or when you cough or sneeze
- a decrease in pain on resting
- pain on breathing deeply.

Because most of us are wary of chest pains, the condition can be scary. It doesn't help that costochrondritis pains are most commonly felt on the left side of the chest – although they can be just on the right side, or even both sides. If you are ever truly concerned that you are having a heart attack, get immediate medical help. It's better to be safe than sorry.

Mitral valve prolapse

Another condition common to people with fibromyalgia is mitral valve prolapse, and this can contribute to chest wall pain. The mitral valve is one of the heart valves, and when it bulges significantly during heartbeats, it is said to have 'prolapsed'. Although this sounds rather serious, it is normally a benign condition that can be easily diagnosed and requires no treatment. Very occasionally, the condition is more severe and causes a rapid irregular heartbeat, shortness of breath and other cardiac problems. If you experience any of the aforementioned symptoms, you should seek medical attention immediately.

Jaw pain

About one in three people with fibromyalgia have long-standing jaw and face pain, known medically as temperomandibular jaw dysfunction, or TMJD. In TMJD, there are no problems within the joint itself, but the muscles and ligaments in and around the joint have become taut and inflamed, causing pain and numbness. On chewing there is often a cracking or crunching sound; it can be uncomfortable to bite and some people have difficulty even opening their mouths. The condition is often triggered by traumatic impact of some kind, or even by prolonged dental work.

The following symptoms can occur with TMJD, although they are rarely present all at once:

- pains that vary between aching and stabbing in the face and jaw
- difficulty opening your mouth
- ringing in the ears (tinnitus)
- numbness in the areas affected
- dizziness.

Less common symptoms include the following:

- facial twitching
- flushing (reddening) of the face
- swollen and inflamed feeling in the jaw.

A specially made splint, worn over the lower teeth in bed at night, can improve the situation, as can a painkilling injection into the joint. Such an injection cured my own TMJD, but I am careful to avoid hard or chewy foods as I wouldn't wish it to come back. See your dentist if you would like to try a splint, or your doctor if you prefer to discuss the possibility of having a painkilling injection.

Numbness and tingling

Known as 'parasthesia', numbness and tingling usually occur in the fingers and toes. Paresthesia may be a symptom of any one of several different conditions and should always be reported to your doctor. When all else is ruled out, it will then be put down as a quirk of your fibromyalgia, a sign that soft tissue problems are interfering with the normal transmission of nerve messages.

Restless leg syndrome

Studies have indicated that people with fibromyalgia are about 11 times more likely than healthy people to have restless leg syndrome (RLS). RLS is a sleep-related movement disorder in which you have an irresistible urge to move your legs in bed. People with RLS experience creeping sensations, accompanied sometimes by twitching, tingling, itching, prickling or aching, in their legs, which is temporarily relieved by moving them. The sensations soon return and so you move your legs once more. This makes it difficult to fall asleep and may cause you to wake a lot during the night. I have RLS, and often don't realize how much my legs are aching until I lie down in bed at night. I constantly have the urge to move my legs to get some ease, but it's not until I massage them and walk around that I get some benefit. I don't have the twitching, tingling and so on, just the troublesome aching that demands relief.

RLS is thought to be the result of anaemia caused by iron or folic acid deficiency. There may also be a genetic link as the condition often runs in families. Some medications can make RLS worse – antidepressants, calcium blockers, most anti-nausea medications and some anti-allergy drugs. Caffeine is also known to worsen the condition.

You can improve RLS by including adequate iron, folic acid, calcium, potassium and magnesium in your diet. It is best also to cut down on stimulants such as caffeine, nicotine and alcohol. Drinking plenty of water can be helpful, too. As low blood sugar may play a part in RLS, have a light, slow-release snack, such as a yogurt, low-fat cheese or oatcakes, before going to bed. Taking up yoga can be helpful, too. If you can't get to sleep for the problem, try massaging your legs then walking around for a few minutes.

See your doctor if you think you have RLS. There is an excellent drug called Pramipexole, a dopamine receptor agonist, which works very well for most people. It can also help to improve sleep problems.

Sjögren's syndrome – dry eyes and mouth

About a third of all fibromyalgia patients report dry, gritty eyes, a dry mouth and dry lips – a condition known as Sjögren's syndrome. This is most common in women aged 40 to 60, and results from the immune system attacking and damaging tear and saliva glands. The eyes can itch and burn, which is very uncomfortable; it makes wearing normal contact lenses difficult, or impossible. As the condition progresses, other organs of the body can be affected, such as the skin, internal organs, a woman's vagina, and so on. The condition can even cause fatigue – unfortunately on top of the fatigue already experienced in fibromyalgia.

A dry mouth can make speech and swallowing difficult and the discomfort is so great that some people need to constantly hydrate themselves. A friend of mine has had to start wearing false teeth as a result of her Sjögren's syndrome; the condition caused her to gradually lose her own.

If you have Sjögren's syndrome, your doctor may prescribe anti-inflammatory drugs or an immune system suppressant. As yet, little else can be done by the medical profession. However, a number of natural treatments are now helping many people.

- Preliminary evidence shows that oral hygiene products containing bovine colostrum (colostrum from cows) can be beneficial.
- Toothpaste containing a substance called betaine may help.
- Gamma-linolenic acid (GLA), an essential fatty acid in the omega 6 family, may improve the dry eyes and fatigue associated with Sjögren's syndrome.
- Studies of flaxseed oil have also shown promising results for the treatment of this condition.
- Artificial teardrops, which may ease the itching and help prevent painful reddening, can be purchased over the counter from pharmacies.
- Vaginal lubricants, such as KY gel, can be very useful.
- The supplement N-acetyl cysteine (NAC), a modified form of the amino acid cysteine, when taken orally is thought to help loosen secretions. This supplement is available from some health food shops and websites. In a small trial, taking 200mg of NAC three times daily improved eye-related symptoms and showed promise for mouth-related symptoms. A much larger trial is required for more conclusive results.
- If you wear normal contact lenses but can't cope with them

because of sore eyes, special contact lenses are now available for dry eyes – and they are noted as being comfortable.

Reynaud's syndrome

The hypersensitive nervous system in fibromyalgia can give rise to Reynaud's syndrome. This condition is usually triggered by cold temperatures, and describes a sudden restriction of blood flow to the extremities, making the area turn white. Indeed, cold temperatures can produce a temporary spasm in the fingers or toes, which makes the small blood vessels narrow and limit blood flow. The fingers and toes are most commonly affected, but it can also occur in the ears and nose. Stress can trigger the onset of a Reynaud's syndrome spasm, as the stress response automatically causes blood vessels to restrict.

I don't have this syndrome myself, but I well remember the intense pain I felt as a child on heating up icy cold hands after playing in the snow – my family called the pain 'hot aches'. It is identical to the pain experienced by people with Reynaud's on a regular basis, as the blood begins to flow back into the affected areas. Some people have near continual Reynaud's attacks, even in warmer weather or when they're not particularly stressed.

You can do the following to help prevent attacks:

- Avoid exposure to the cold.
- Wear gloves, if necessary even when removing something from the fridge or freezer.
- On cold days, layer your clothing to trap in the heat.
- Boost your circulation by being as active as possible.
- Have at least two hot meals a day.
- Control your stress levels by pacing yourself and using relaxation techniques.
- Eat plenty of fruit and vegetables – vitamins C and E can help strengthen blood vessels.
- Take the supplement ginkgo biloba to boost your blood circulation.
- Include several helpings of oily fish a week in your diet and take fish oil capsules to raise levels of prostacyclin, a substance that helps to keep blood vessels dilated and is believed to be lacking in people with Reynaud's.

Pain on sexual intercourse

In women, pain or discomfort during sexual intercourse is called dyspareunia. The pain can be so severe that sex is not feasible, perhaps to the detriment of the relationship. The condition is thought to be part of the increased sensitivity to pain that comes with fibromyalgia. However, it is important that you inform your doctor about it, as dyspareunia is sometimes caused by a bacterial infection or trauma to the pelvic or vaginal area. Tests will be carried out and treatment offered, if appropriate.

If dyspareunia is a part of your fibromyalgia, you stand the best chance of overcoming or at least reducing the problem if you can improve your general health. Indeed, those who work hard at improving their condition and succeed in living a fairly active and fulfilling life are often able to start having pain-free sexual intercourse once more.

Painful menstrual cramps

The lowered pain threshold and increased pain sensitivity that come with fibromyalgia can even create painful periods in women, a condition known as dysmenorrhoea. In fact, up to 90 per cent of women with fibromyalgia have a lot of discomfort during menstruation, and approximately 45 per cent have dysmenorrhoea. The condition is characterized by severe abdominal cramps, pelvic pain and lower back pain during the menstrual cycle. The cramping pains can be so severe that the woman is confined to the house for the first few days of her period, or even bed-bound. Most women with fibromyalgia who have dysmenorrhoea have had pain-free periods earlier in their lives.

Symptoms linked to dysmenorrhoea include the following:

- moderate to severe abdominal cramping
- shooting pains in the abdomen, going into your lower back and thighs
- cold sweats
- dizziness and fainting
- headache
- nausea
- diarrhoea
- fatigue

- nervous irritability
- exacerbation of other fibromyalgia symptoms.

Don't be embarrassed to go and see your doctor if your periods are excessively painful and you experience any of the above symptoms of dysmenorrhoea. Doctors are well acquainted with 'intimate' problems and can offer useful treatment, such as anti-prostaglandin medication (prostaglandins are the hormones released by the uterus to make it contract). Studies have shown that anti-prostaglandin medication helps in an impressive 80 per cent of cases. Other medications such as NSAIDs can reduce the cramping pains.

Skin problems

A substantial 70 to 80 per cent of people with fibromyalgia have associated skin problems, in the form of dryness, flaking, mottling, itchiness and rashes. The following are common possible skin problems and their causes.

- *Dryness* – many people with fibromyalgia have permanently dry, cracked skin, anywhere on the body, and the damaged skin can peel, which causes discomfort. The hands and fingers are most commonly affected. In some people, skin dryness, flaking and cracking may be a manifestation of Sjögren's syndrome (see page 70).
- *Itchiness and rashes* – very common in fibromyalgia, itchy skin can cause rashes (in the form of raised scaly bumps) all over the body. Over-scratching can then lead to soreness and infection. Most itchiness is thought to result from misunderstood pain signals.
- *Mottling* – sometimes skin discolouration and random dark spots can develop, particularly on the inside of the forearms and thighs. Sun exposure can further darken the spots or make them red and swollen. The cause of this is an overactive pituitary gland, the area of the brain responsible for producing melanin. Melanin is the substance that creates the colour pigment in our eyes, skin and hair – the more melanin there is, the darker the colour. When the pituitary gland produces too much melanin, as it occasionally does in fibromyalgia, the excess spills over into the skin, causing the dark spots.

Treatments

First of all, visit your doctor if you are troubled by skin problems. If you have dry skin, you are likely to be prescribed an excellent corticosteroid cream which should calm the itch and prevent rashes developing. You can also buy heavy creams and moisturizers over the counter to apply liberally every day.

It is best to treat a non-infectious skin rash with over-the-counter hydrocortisone cream, used for one week. If the rash persists, your doctor will probably prescribe an appropriate cream. For mottled skin, your doctor may either recommend a bleaching cream or refer you for a few sessions of ultraviolet light therapy at your local hospital.

Visual problems

In fibromyalgia, the eyes are normally quite sensitive to smoke and very dry air, among other things. The result can be pain, blurred vision and watering. Irritated eye muscles easily become painful and even go into spasm, which makes focusing difficult.

Visual overload is also common in fibromyalgia. The messages from our eyes sometimes jumble in our brains, making our minds go quite blank for a second or two. I often find it difficult to recognize faces; as I live where there are usually crowds of holidaymakers, I believe that my problem is caused by visual overload.

Fortunately, the visual problems in fibromyalgia do not lead to more significant problems, such as glaucoma or detached retina.

6

Other things you can do to help yourself

When illness enters your life, it's not unusual to believe that your only option is drug treatment – taking the medications recommended by your doctor. However, if you treated fibromyalgia solely with medications, you would not improve past a certain point, for no drug or drug combination can yet lead to full recovery.

Fibromyalgia responds best to a multi-faceted treatment approach, incorporating exercise, diet, stress control and so on, which should greatly improve your health and emotional wellbeing. The multi-faceted approach is described in this chapter.

Exercise

I have chosen to begin with exercise as this is the great bugbear, to put it mildly, in fibromyalgia self-treatment. We know how important exercise is, for we are constantly told so, but trying to carry out an exercise regime can be the stuff of nightmares. Oh, we start out with the very best of intentions and the determination to gradually build up the routine and number of repetitions, but we rapidly become unstuck when our first venture brings on agonies so great, the last thing we want is to risk them again.

The majority of people can see no further than the pain each attempt at exercise brings, which of course is understandable. The everyday pain of fibromyalgia is challenging enough, and to risk greatly exacerbating that is contrary to human nature. It's no wonder, then, that many people believe that an exercise routine equates to added pain, and dare not risk putting themselves through it. I must 'bang the exercise drum' myself, though, for not exercising at all is hardly the answer. In fibromyalgia, our muscles are invariably tight and out of condition, and the very best way to stretch and strengthen them is to submit them to a daily exercise routine. Without regular exercise our bodies are liable to become ever more painful. Indeed, evidence suggests that sedentary people with fibromyalgia have rather more pain than their exercising counterparts. Avoiding exercise can even lead to other diseases, such as osteoporosis, diabetes and cardiovascular problems.

Exercise can even stave off fibromyalgia

People whose fibromyalgia was triggered by a physical trauma, such as a whiplash injury, report that their activity levels were, probably for reasons of self-protection, reduced significantly after the trauma. This is what happened in my case, and I can't help wondering what the outcome might have been if, in the years after the trauma and before fibromyalgia set in, I had asked my doctor to refer me for physiotherapy, where I would have been taught a series of stretching and strengthening exercises.

If you have experienced a trauma but don't have full-blown fibromyalgia, you may be able to ward it off by taking up gentle daily exercise to strengthen the damaged tissues. Ask your doctor about the possibility of a referral for physiotherapy, where you can start doing the best exercises for your particular case.

Exercising without added pain

There is a secret, a trick to exercising without added pain – and it's a very simple one. All it requires is a gradual, inch-by-inch start, and the recognition that you must stop the moment you feel the slightest increase in discomfort or pain. It demands that you rest sufficiently after exercising to allow your body to recover – even if only a couple of head turns and arm stretches have been completed. For some it can take months or even years to accomplish a reasonable daily stretching routine of, say, ten minutes in duration.

Although the solution in itself is simple, I realize that it's not so easy to put into practice. It takes a lot of patience and self-discipline to allow yourself to go only so far every day, to know that you can do only so much and no more. You will be so pleased that you bothered to be super-careful, though, when you start to feel stronger, more energized and more mobile; you may notice a difference in only a few weeks.

Knowing when to incorporate a little more into your routine at each 'stage' is always a tricky one – 'stages' being the occasions when you feel strong enough to add further repetitions or movements. It's best to increase by only one or two repetitions at each stage and to proceed as carefully as possible.

A personalized routine

As pain levels fluctuate considerably in fibromyalgia, it is important to develop a routine tailored to your particular strengths and weaknesses. Many books of exercises are available, including my own *Living with Fibromyalgia*, in which series of diagrams outline each particular exercise action.

Pick out any exercises that you think you can comfortably do, and write a brief description of each one on a sheet of paper – this is your 'starter' routine. Now fix the sheet of paper to a door or wall near to your planned exercise area, and promise yourself that you will incorporate exercise into your life, from now on. As I've mentioned, only gentle stretches may be within your scope at the outset, but you should later be able to expand your routine.

On the first day of your exercise routine, remember to avoid pushing yourself – even a little tightening of the muscles can translate into soreness later on. Ideally, when you finish your routine, you should feel as if you could have done more. Some discomfort may arise later, but this is fine so long as it 'rests off' during the subsequent few hours. If there is still added discomfort, or even pain, the next day (on top of what you would normally expect to have), either your chosen routine was too ambitious or you did not relax enough afterwards and allow sufficient time for your body to recover. Give yourself two or three further relaxing days, or until all the additional pain has disappeared, then recommence your exercising with more a basic routine, and make sure you rest sufficiently afterwards. Bear in mind that you should be able to include all exercises you have dropped when your body is stronger.

People with milder symptoms (or individuals who have worked hard to reduce symptoms that were originally severe) may wish to try using an item called a theraband – a long elasticated strip that can be manipulated in a number of ways to give your body a workout. The large inflatable Swiss ball is also now popular as an exercise device. Stretch over the ball, moving back and forth to help massage tight muscles. As always, with whatever exercise you choose to do, start out carefully, rest enough afterwards, and try building up very slowly.

Aerobic exercise

Please don't faint at the thought of doing aerobic exercise! You don't *have* to do anything, only what your body tells you it can manage – but that may be a little more than you realize, especially after you have been carrying out stretches for a few months or more.

Low-impact aerobic exercise can:

- prevent muscle wastage (atrophy);
- promote blood circulation, so bringing oxygen and nutrients to the muscles and other connective tissues;
- boost strength and endurance;
- strengthen the heart and lungs.

As well as the above, aerobic exercise should result in less general hurting and a better quality of life. In fibromyalgia, the exercises should be at a low to moderate intensity and should raise your heart rate slightly, causing you to breathe harder and faster. The movements are usually rhythmical, using the large muscles in the legs and buttocks. Examples include walking (either outside or on a treadmill), trampoline jogging (using a small fitness trampoline), cycling (either outside or on a static exercise bike indoors), swimming, and using exercise equipment such as a cross-country ski-machine. Jogging is usually too demanding for people with fibromyalgia.

Take aerobic exercise extremely slowly, and gradually build up your tolerance. It's also important to find an activity you enjoy, so you are more likely to do it on a regular basis.

Pacing

Pacing requires that you plan every day of your life, for as long as pain is a problem. If you already use pacing, you'll know what a useful technique it is. If you haven't yet tried it, I urge you to do so. Pacing reduces the frequency of flare-ups and leads to gradual improvement, especially if you are also using exercise, improved diet and so on. In my opinion, if you were able to select only one of the strategies described in this chapter, I would strongly recommend that it be pacing. It's *that* important.

When you have fibromyalgia, the symptoms can fluctuate so much, it is like spending your life on a rollercoaster. You are likely to career between troublesome periods and relatively smoother times. The latter tend not to last very long, however – when the going is good it's always tempting to push yourself too far, with the result that you come to a full stop and need a great deal of rest. The cycle of overactivity followed by flare-ups, then extensive rest, is anxiety-provoking and thoroughly demoralizing, making you feel out of control.

Pacing involves not doing any type of activity, or resting, for too long. It is an energy and lifestyle management strategy through which people with chronic pain can stabilize their symptoms and so start to make real progress. Using this strategy often means that the rhythm of overactivity followed by setbacks can be overcome, and you learn to live within the limitations imposed by your current state of health. Try always to alternate activity and rest periods, with the aim of gradually increasing your 'up and about' time and reducing your 'down' time.

Pacing not only enables you to get stronger, it also leads to a significant reduction in levels of stress. It allows the rollercoaster car you are in to leave the extreme ups and downs of its normal track and begin gliding smoothly along a road with only gentle undulations. And without the twists, turns, bumps and thuds, you feel far more content. It can be said, then, that symptom stability greatly encourages emotional stability.

Of course, pacing is just common sense. It simply means taking planned breaks and listening to your body. It's unfortunate, though, that people with fibromyalgia sometimes either lose confidence in this ability, or experience greatly delayed pain, and both of these make pacing difficult.

Swap activity types

It is important that any activity – whether it requires physical, social, mental or emotional effort – is split into manageable portions or tasks; and having achieved one task, if you have retained some energy and are not hurting more than normal, you can switch from one type of activity to another before taking a planned rest. Of course, swapping one activity for another is not always feasible, especially if you are trying to do something time-consuming like going to the shops. However, switching activity types, at least on some occasions, can postpone further tiredness and pain.

Planning your everyday life

Planning is essential to effective pacing. Below is an example of a daily routine plan for someone who doesn't go out to work but is well enough to deal with light chores. Of course, you must take your current state of health into account when formulating your own daily plan. You may not be able to do half as much as in the example shown here, so your plan will reflect this – or you may be able to do more.

Living according to a plan may seem artificial – but it gives you back the sense of being in control, which is enormously lifting. Changing to a planned life rather than pushing ahead and reacting to symptoms is well worth it when you find yourself with less pain and more energy. Pacing also allows you to understand the cycle of flare-ups followed by enforced rest. People with fibromyalgia often view their ups and downs as random – a peculiarity of their illness – but living life according to a plan helps us to see that flare-ups generally arise in response to overexertion.

Example of a daily routine pacing plan

7.30–8.30	Get up, get washed, get dressed, have breakfast.
8.30–8.45	Carry out your chosen exercise routine.
8.45–9.30	Lie on your bed and listen to music or perform a relaxation routine.
9.30–10.30	Deal with your emails, perhaps play a computer game.
10.30–11.00	Do some light dusting and tidying up.
11.00–12.00	Lie on the sofa and listen to the radio or a radio download on an MP3 player.
12.00–12.45	Prepare and eat a light lunch.
12.45–13.30	Walk to the local shop for a few light items.
13.30–14.30	Read a book.
14.30–15.30	Prepare meat and vegetables for a casserole; put in the oven to slow cook.
16.00–17.30	Lie on your bed. Practise relaxation or listen to an audio book.
17.30–18.30	Welcome your partner home, and serve and eat your evening meal.
18.30–19.30	Lie on the sofa to watch television, while your partner washes up.
19.30–20.30	Spend time chatting with your partner.
20.30–21.30	Watch television, listen to the radio, read a book or play a board game.
21.30–22.00	Relax in a hot bath with aromatherapy oils or Epsom salts.
22.00–22.30	Go to bed, perhaps listening to a relaxation CD until sleepy.

Delayed pain

The onset of pain is a stark warning to healthy people that they need to slow down; but in fibromyalgia pain in response to activity can be delayed. For instance, you may experience no rise in symptoms when you are out doing the shopping, but three or four hours later your shoulder and arm may be aching badly. If your pain is so delayed that it doesn't alert you to a particular overexertion, the pacing technique is your best chance of making a significant improvement.

Be prepared to alter your plan

You will probably need to make constant alterations to your pacing plan, depending on your responses to different activities. For instance, if you find that reading a book for an hour makes your neck and shoulder muscles tighten and ache, find a more comfortable position for reading, or reduce your reading time.

Listen to your body

If your pain is not normally delayed, take great care: at the first signs of tightening or rising discomfort, stop what you are doing and have a relaxing break, whether or not you are close to finishing what you are doing. If you live with a certain level of pain all the time, you should stop the moment the pain increases, if not before that point. It's no good being aware that the pain is worsening if you don't immediately do something about it. Indeed, if you don't act, you will surely fall into a flare-up and need a lot more rest than you had bargained for.

A healthy diet

The best diet for fibromyalgia that I know of is discussed in detail in my book *The Fibromyalgia Healing Diet*. Remember that a healthy diet does not have to be boring or tasteless. Healthy foods can actually be tastier than anything processed, prepackaged or picked up from the local takeaway.

Here is an outline of the most salient points of the fibromyalgia diet:

Fresh fruit and vegetables

People with fibromyalgia tend to have a lot of acid in their bodies. This can be combated by the alkalizing properties of fresh fruit and vegetables, which have a high vitamin and mineral content. Try not to eat too many tomatoes, though, as they are highly acidic.

Select locally grown organic fruit and vegetables that are in season, and it is best to eat as fresh and as raw as possible. When you have to cook your vegetables, use unsalted (or lightly salted) water and simmer for the minimum length of time. Lightly steaming and stir-frying are healthy alternatives. Try out a variety of green salads and eat one every day.

Legumes (peas and beans)

Legumes are cheap to buy and contain large amounts of protein, which is vital to the body for growth and maintenance. Protein also helps to relieve stiffness and pain.

The soya bean is a complete protein, of which there are many derivatives including soya milk, tofu, tempeh and miso. Soya milk can be used as an alternative to cow's milk.

Seeds

Sunflower, sesame, hemp, flax and pumpkin seeds are very important for strengthening the body's systems. They can be eaten as they are as a snack, sprinkled on to salads and cereals, or used in baking.

Nuts

All nuts contain vital nutrients, but almonds, cashews, walnuts, brazils and pecans perhaps offer the greatest array. Eat a wide assortment as snacks, with cereal and in baking. Obviously, if you are allergic to nuts, they must be avoided at all costs.

Grains

Whole-grain and wholemeal flours provide us with the complex unrefined carbohydrates our bodies require – and again, organic is best. Many types of grain are good for us, but wheat – our staple in the west – contains gluten and can be highly allergenic for some people. If you suspect you have a gluten allergy, ask your doctor if you can be properly tested. And although it's nutritious, wheat is acidic and not recommended in fibromyalgia.

With the exception of wheat, aim to consume a variety of grains, including oats, rye, barley (generally available as pearl barley), corn, buckwheat, brown rice and mixed grains. Brown rice, millet, buckwheat and maize/corn are all gluten-free and invaluable to people with a gluten allergy or sensitivity.

Fats and oils

Fats are a great source of essential fatty acids (EFAs), which improve energy levels, blood circulation and oxygen uptake. They also help to boost levels of serotonin, which, as explained earlier, is in short supply in fibromyalgia. Our bodies are unable to manufacture EFAs, so they can only come from our diets.

There are two distinct types of fatty acid – one bad, one good:

- *Saturated fat* – this type of fat should be avoided because of its detrimental effect on the heart and other organs. It comes mainly from animal sources and is generally solid at room temperature. Butter is a valuable source of oils and vitamin A, but should be used sparingly. Margarine contains many additives and is not recommended in fibromyalgia.
- *Unsaturated fat* – also called polyunsaturated or monounsaturated fat, unsaturated fat has a protective effect on the heart and other organs. Omega 3 and omega 6 oils occur naturally in oily fish (such as mackerel, herring, sardines, tuna), nuts and seeds, and are usually liquid at room temperature. Try to eat oily fish at least three times a week and use cold-pressed oil (olive, rapeseed, safflower and sunflower oil) daily, for dressings and in cooking.

Cow's milk products

Cow's milk products include cheese, yogurt, cream, butter, ice cream, condensed milk, evaporated milk and powdered milk, and all are rich in calcium, protein and the vitamins A, D and E. However, little trace of these vitamins remains after the pasteurization process and they are often replaced (fortified) by dairies in harmful amounts. Moreover, cow's milk products contain a lot of the sugar lactose – indeed, a glass of milk contains half as much sugar as in a glass of a fizzy drink. Lactose is difficult for many people to digest and can cause sensitivity problems such as bloating, gas, stomach aches and diarrhoea.

The calcium in cow's milk products is the best thing about it. What you may not know is that sufficient calcium can be obtained from regular consumption of dark leafy vegetables, seaweed (kelp, wakame and hijiki), nuts and seeds, beans, oranges and figs. Children need to drink milk, however.

Eggs

The cholesterol in eggs is not now thought to be a risk factor in arterial disease. Indeed, major new research has shown that egg cholesterol has a clinically insignificant effect on blood cholesterol. Buy free-range eggs and eat them soft-boiled or lightly poached, as a hard yolk will bind the lecithin, which is great at mopping up excess fat.

The Food Standards Agency now states that most people don't need to limit their consumption of eggs so long as they are part of a balanced diet.

Red meat

Red meat usually contains large amounts of saturated fat, so it should be eaten in moderation. Look for organically produced meat, as the use of pesticides, antibiotics and hormones in animal husbandry is an ongoing health issue. If you can't bear to go without red meat, make your serving no larger or thicker than the palm of your hand, and don't eat red meat more than three times a week. Make sure you consume enough other protein in the form of fish, poultry, soya products, cottage cheese, organic live yogurt, nuts, seeds and legumes.

Fish

Fish is particularly beneficial as it is an excellent source of omega 3 fatty acids, amino acids and gamma linoleic acid (GLA), deficiencies of which can aggravate aches and pains. Choose oily cold-water fish, such as sardines, tuna, anchovies, mackerel, trout, salmon, herring (kippers) and pilchards.

Poultry

Chicken and turkey contain far less fat than red meat. They are good sources of protein and essential fatty acids (EFAs), which can improve circulation and oxygen uptake. Try to eat chicken or turkey once or twice a week.

Foods to avoid

Reducing or eliminating the foods mentioned in this section can have a positive effect on your fibromyalgia.

Salt

Because salt can inhibit the growth of harmful micro-organisms, it's added in copious amounts as a preservative to most processed and prepackaged foods. For example, one tin of soup can contain more salt (sodium) than the full recommended daily allowance for an adult. You should try, therefore, to limit your intake of salt in cooking and at the table. If you occasionally buy processed or prepackaged foods, look for 'low salt' or sodium-free' on the label.

Sugar

Sugar consumption has been linked with many disorders, from diabetes to heart disease and cancer. We do need a certain amount of sugar in our diets for conversion to energy, but that can be obtained naturally from fruits and complex carbohydrates.

If you really must sweeten your food and drinks, alternatives to white sugar include raw honey and barley malt. Muscovado and demerara sugars are formed during the early stages of the refining process, and so contain more nutrients than refined white sugar.

Caffeine

Products that contain caffeine – coffee, tea, cocoa, cola drinks, energy drinks and chocolate – affect the adrenal glands and make coping with stress difficult. Consumed regularly in fairly high doses, caffeine is likely to give rise to chronic anxiety (see page 60). My best advice is to remove caffeine products from your diet.

Coffee, tea, cocoa and cola drinks can be replaced by carob, fruit juices, vegetable juices, herbal teas, green tea and redbush tea. Many decaffeinated products don't make a good alternative – they are processed with the use of chemicals. Drink them only in moderation.

Other stimulants to avoid

When fibromyalgia makes you feel low and worn out, your body demands a boost of energy – a 'lift'. However, the lift obtained from a stimulant is short-lived – unlike the damage it can do to your adrenal glands, which are already weakened in fibromyalgia. Stimulants can also lead to or worsen chronic anxiety, low energy and nerve cell damage.

Try to completely eliminate stimulants from your diet, or at least reduce them as much as possible – it *will* make a difference.

Alcohol

Many people with fibromyalgia cannot tolerate alcohol; some say that it causes their blood to run like acid through their veins – this can be how it feels to me, too. According to preliminary studies, the fibromyalgia patients who drink the most alcohol often have the most severe symptoms.

Smoking

If you smoke, you don't need me or anyone else to tell you it's not good for you. What you may not know is that smoking is particularly harmful in fibromyalgia because our central nervous systems are hypersensitive to chemicals. And shockingly, with each inhalation of a cigarette, a massive 600 toxic chemicals are absorbed into the bloodstream. To be blunt, there's little hope of symptom stability if you continue to introduce chemicals into your body.

If you feel that smoking helps you to deal with the stress of the condition, remind yourself that when compared with the damage it does to your health, the trade-off has a very high price.

The food elimination diet

Although most adverse food reactions are due to 'intolerance', we tend to think of all reactions as 'allergies'. An allergy, however, provokes an immediate reaction, varying from a headache to anaphylactic shock – a life-threatening condition – whereas an intolerance reaction can take up to 24 hours to present itself.

Food elimination

You may already have a fairly good idea which foods your body objects to. If not, you can narrow it down by keeping a careful record of all you eat and noting any reactions. When you have a clearer idea of the culprits, eliminate them from your diet for a period of one month. Try to ensure that your diet is still balanced, however.

If you suspect that you are sensitive to several foods, ask your doctor to refer you to an allergy testing clinic. There are many allergy-friendly foods and supplements available from health food shops and pharmacies.

When the offending foods are first withdrawn, you may occasionally experience a withdrawal reaction, producing such symptoms as fatigue, headaches, twitching, and irritability for up to 15 days. Drinking as much water as possible will help to reduce these symptoms.

Reintroduction strategy

Towards the end of the month you may feel better than you have for a long time. The feeling of well-being can be so great that you won't want to bother reintroducing the excluded foods. But if you do wish to start eating them again, do it carefully by following the procedure below:

- *Day 1*: In the morning, reintroduce a small amount of one of the eliminated foods (not a full-sized portion). Do the same later in the day and record any symptoms.
- *Day 2*: If you had no adverse reaction, repeat the exercise. Once again, record any symptoms experienced. If you get through the second day, this is really good news!
- *Days 3–4*: Wait for two further days before you can safely reintroduce this food into your diet on a regular basis.

Repeat this four-day reintroduction procedure with each food eliminated. Any side effects should have occurred within these four days. If you do experience symptoms – for example, if you develop a headache after reintroducing mushrooms – it would be better to leave that food alone for at least six months before trying them again. Some foods may always trigger adverse reactions and it is best to withdraw them from your diet altogether.

You may be disappointed, too, if your problem is true allergy. The offending food will provoke an immediate reaction – your immune system responds as if it is being invaded, setting up antibodies to the food in question. Obviously you will need to continue avoiding this food. Dairy products are the top food allergen, and wheat the second. If you are sensitive to either of these (or both), make sure you replace them with plenty of protein and oil-containing foods and/or alternative grains.

Nutritional supplements

You may have heard some doctors say that it's not necessary for people to take nutritional supplements, and we obtain sufficient nutrients from the foods we eat. This is usually true if you are fit and healthy, but if you have an illness of some kind you are naturally deficient in certain vitamins and minerals. Making no effort to put back these nutrients means that you are likely to slow down your rate of improvement. A healthy balanced diet will restock your body with essential nutrients, but unfortunately there may always be a shortfall. Experts in chronic illness are therefore still advocating the use of certain supplements.

Vitamin and mineral supplements

- *Vitamin C (ascorbic acid)* – in fibromyalgia there is a shortfall of ascorbic acid. This vitamin is an excellent detoxifier and helps to reduce stress. Take up to 3,000mg of vitamin C daily.
- *Vitamin B complex* – as the B group of vitamins helps to reduce anxiety and stress, it is best to take a high potency B complex supplement twice daily.
- *Vitamin E* – vitamin E helps to improve sleep, alleviate fatigue, boost healing and aid in the utilization of vitamin A by the body. You can take up to 400IU daily.
- *Vitamin A (beta-carotene, the precursor to retinol)* – this vitamin is necessary for the growth and repair of all bodily tissues. Take up to 10,000 IUs per day.
- *NADH (beta-nicotinamide adenine dinucleotide)* – this co-enzyme enables the body to increase adenosine triphosphate (ATP), the fuel that provides the body with energy. Take 15–30mg daily, depending upon the severity of your symptoms. The dosage should be reduced to 5mg per day when your symptoms improve.
- *Calcium* – this mineral works with magnesium to ensure proper muscle contraction/relaxations, and is important to good nervous system function. Take up to 1,000mg daily.
- *Magnesium* – as magnesium deficiency is universal in fibromyalgia, supplementation is highly recommended. This mineral is important for the absorption of many vitamins and minerals, and it aids the conversion of blood sugar to energy. Take 600–1,200mg daily.
- *Manganese* – this mineral plays a vital role in fibromyalgia, helping to create energy from glucose and aiding in the normalization of the central nervous system. Take up to 10mg daily.
- *Zinc* – digestion, protein synthesis and good immune system function require plenty of zinc. Take up to 15mg daily.
- *Potassium* – this mineral works with sodium to regulate heart and muscle function. It also helps to ensure a correct acid/alkaline balance, and the normal transmission of nerve impulses. Take up to 5,000mg daily.

Other useful supplements

- *Malic acid* – this supplement plays a vital role in the operation of the 'malic acid shuttle service', which delivers important nutrients to the cells for conversion to energy. It is particularly effective when combined with magnesium. Some supplement manufacturers now offer magnesium malate, which combines the two. Take up to 200mg daily.

- *Co-enzyme Q10 (CoQ10)* – this enzyme is important in fibromyalgia as it helps to increase mental and physical energy and alleviate pain and fatigue. It works by aiding the transfer of oxygen and energy between components of the cells and between the blood and the tissues. Take up to 100mg daily.
- *Boron* – this trace element is important to maintaining good muscular health. Because people with fibromyalgia may be inactive for long periods, it can also help to reduce calcium loss from the bones. Take up to 3mg daily.
- *5-hydroxytryptophan* (5-HTP) – because of its ability to increase serotonin levels, this phytonutrient (plant derivative) is useful in fibromyalgia for promoting sleep and reducing pain, anxiety and fatigue. The RDA for fibromyalgia is 100–500mg daily, depending upon the severity of symptoms.

Begin by taking vitamins A, C and E (known as the ACE vitamins), together with CoQ10, zinc and manganese supplements, which work as fine antioxidants, reducing the oxidative stress of fibromyalgia and aiding the healing process. These substances may be purchased together in a single antioxidant supplement from certain health supplement manufacturers. Alternatively, the constituents may be bought separately, but generally at a higher price.

After one month of taking these vitamins and antioxidants, I suggest that you add magnesium and malic acid supplementation. These nutrients work together to reduce pain, fatigue and low muscle stamina, but can generally only be bought separately. A multi-mineral supplement containing calcium, manganese, zinc, boron and magnesium should also be taken.

During the next month, you can start taking another of the recommended supplements, depending upon your choice. They all work in different ways to improve fibromyalgia. I appreciate that a fair amount of expenditure is called for – but because of the many deficiencies in fibromyalgia, supplementation is important. Having said that, please remember that taking only one or two supplements is better than taking none at all. The antioxidant supplements are of prime importance, as is the magnesium/malic acid (magnesium malate) supplement.

The dosages should be reduced to maintenance levels after eight to ten months.

Whether you go on to take any of the other supplements mentioned is entirely your choice, and perhaps dependent upon your finances.

It is best to consult your doctor before embarking on a course of nutritional supplements. Some of them interact with certain medications, and so may adversely affect particular medical conditions.

Address your stress

What some experts refer to as a 'period of catastrophic stress' can actually change your hormonal status and lead to fibromyalgia. And when you have fibromyalgia, ongoing stress or new episodes of stress can cause symptom flare-ups. An individual who feels continually stressed, because of either unfortunate life events or their personality type, is likely to have repeated flare-ups and a gradual worsening of their overall condition.

Inflammatory blood cells (cytokines) and stress

The hormones involved in stress are known to affect the balance of our inflammatory white blood cells, known as cytokines. Recent studies have shown that people with fibromyalgia have above average levels of these cytokines – and unfortunately, the more we have, the more we hurt. This means that a pain that feels moderate to a person with normal cytokine levels could easily feel severe to someone with fibromyalgia. The answer here is to work at lowering your stress levels, which will then automatically lower levels of cytokines.

Ongoing stressful situations

There are plenty of people who find themselves, through no fault of their own, in a life situation that creates a lot of anxiety and stress. Your child may be ill or handicapped in some way, your elderly parent may rely on you for help and support, or your partner doesn't accept that you're ill and generally treats you quite badly.

It's common for a person with fibromyalgia to endure a stressful situation for years or even decades. And all the time, their fibromyalgia is getting worse, making them less physically and emotionally able to cope. If this applies to you, there is bound to be a point where you say enough is enough and you have to step back from the situation, perhaps passing over the reins to another, more capable person or body of people.

However much you love a handicapped child, it's very stressful too. My own brother was born with brain damage and my parents were continually overwrought by his erratic behaviour; they worried that his condition would worsen and were fearful of what would become of him. For years they struggled to cope with the situation, until my mother's blood pressure rose startlingly high and my father's heart began to fail. At last, when my brother was in his mid-forties, my husband and I suggested that he buy a little house very close to them, to allow them time to relax and unwind. They were sure that my brother wouldn't cope, but they were in for a real surprise. They continued to deal with his paperwork, his ironing and cleaning, but he was able to feed himself. My mother had, very painstakingly, taught him to cook a basic roast dinner, and so every Sunday he piled high five plates of food to microwave during the week. So not only were my parents able to relax more, my brother felt proud as punch that he was living on his own, and that did him the world of good. Sadly, my father died suddenly a year after my brother moved out, but my mother always says that that last year together was the best they ever had. I can't help thinking that if they had made those changes a decade or so earlier, my father might then not have become so ill.

In today's world, the social services system can be a great boon to people with 'learning difficulties' – and to their families, of course. For instance, there are day centres that provide transport each way, care can be obtained in the home, respite care can give families a break, and so on. If you have a child who is disabled in some way, aim to get all the help you can. The same goes for those who are the main carer of an elderly relative. If other family members are in the picture, don't hesitate to ask for their help, too.

Having a partner who doesn't understand your condition can be very frustrating. It makes you feel unloved, disrespected and generally sad. If he or she is good for you in every other way, it's worth making a big effort to help them grasp the situation. I once read an excellent article in *FaMily* (the magazine of the UK Fibromyalgia organization) about a person with chronic illness who gave her friend ten spoons, explaining that each spoon resembled the amount of effort (in terms of pain and exhaustion) it took to perform an action. For instance, in one day, if she had ten spoons to start with, it took her two spoons to get showered and dressed, one spoon to make and eat breakfast, one to check her emails, two to drive her car to the shops and two to carry shopping. By late afternoon in the hypothetical day, the friend had only one spoon left to hand over – but cooking a meal would take two spoons, as would washing up afterwards. She had no option but to make beans on toast, then, as all her spoons were used up, go to bed. Perhaps this little bit of play-acting would work with your partner, or another person who doesn't understand.

Demonstrating the fact that you must pay a price for everything you do can really get through. The other person will, hopefully, realize how important it is that you pick and choose your activities and that you have to pace yourself carefully to get through the day. As to trying the spoon method, remember that some people have more 'spoons' than others. Be careful to assess beforehand how many 'spoons' you have – how many you can use in a day without overdoing it.

If your partner is generally unsupportive, not just where your illness is concerned, I doubt, in truth, that you will be able to change the situation. You need, then, to assess whether the relationship is causing you too much stress or whether you would be more stressed on your own, and for emotional reasons rather than practical ones. Often the thought of splitting up is far worse than the reality, where a poor relationship is concerned. If you are very disabled, you will need to organize support for yourself, from the social services to your family and friends. Taking that leap into single life is difficult for anyone and you will almost certainly endure extra flare-ups for a while. But once your life is on more of an even keel you are likely to wish that you had taken action a long time earlier.

A stress-reducing tip

When things get too much for you, stop what you are doing and mentally stand back from the situation. Breathe right down into your abdomen, deeply, but gently, making sure that your 'out' breath is longer than your 'in' breath. During the out breath, say to yourself, slowly, 'Relax'. Repeat the exercise until you feel calmer. This really works!

Relaxation

Being able to relax helps you to manage your fibromyalgia. Here is a simple relaxation technique: awareness meditation. Another method of relaxation is the deep breathing technique (see pages 93–4).

Awareness meditation

Relaxing without closing your eyes is known as 'awareness meditation'. The term relates to the state of being aware of your life and surroundings while at the same time entering a deeply relaxed place. Here is what you do.

1 Go into a warm room where you know you won't be disturbed for as long as you need to rest and relax. Make sure that the room is not too bright. (You may need to draw the curtains or switch on a small table lamp to create a restful atmosphere.)
2 Lie on your back on a supportive surface – perhaps a bed with an orthopaedic mattress. Make yourself comfortable.
3 Purposefully relax all your muscles, starting at the top with your face and neck and ending with your feet and toes.
4 Don't look around too much. If you like, try to focus loosely on one particular object without actually thinking about it. You will get better at this with practice.
5 As thoughts pass through your mind, don't hang on to them. Simply allow them to float away. If there is a problem in your life at the moment, don't pay attention to it. Once again, practice should make this skill second nature.
6 Stay in the same general position. If you start fidgeting or changing position it's usually because you are focusing on something. If this is so, relax all your muscles once more and allow your conscious mind to drift.
7 If a noise of some kind is likely to disturb your relaxation, wear earplugs or listen to calming music through headphones. Using tape cassettes, CDs or MP3 players is better than listening to the radio, especially if the radio station you normally listen to has advertisements.
8 If your eyelids start to feel droopy, open them, loosely focus again on an object and recommence the whole process. If you sometimes fall asleep during this procedure, it's okay, so long as you are able to sleep at night. However, if you have difficulty sleeping or wake in the morning feeling unrefreshed, having taken naps during the day, make a conscious effort not to drop off.

The deep breathing technique

The chronic stress so common in fibromyalgia can not only lead to flare-ups, it can cause nerviness, hypertension, irritability and depression. It's wise, then, to perform a deep breathing exercise at least once a day.

Deep breathing

In normal breathing, we take oxygen from the atmosphere down into our lungs. The diaphragm contracts and air is pulled into the chest cavity. When we breathe out, we expel carbon dioxide and other waste gases back into the atmosphere. But when we are stressed or upset, we tend to use the rib muscles to expand the chest. We breathe more quickly, sucking in shallowly. This is excellent in a crisis as it allows us to obtain the optimum amount of oxygen in the shortest possible time, providing our bodies with the extra power needed to handle the emergency.

Some people tend to get stuck in chest-breathing mode, however. Long-term shallow breathing is detrimental to physical and emotional health; it can also lead to hyperventilation, panic attacks, chest pains, dizziness and gastro-intestinal problems.

A breathing exercise

Start by carrying out the instructions 1–6 given for awareness meditation (above), except that you should close your eyes. Follow the remaining instructions below.

1 Gradually slow down your breathing, inhaling and exhaling as evenly as possible.
2 Place one hand on your chest and the other on your abdomen, just below your ribcage.
3 As you inhale, allow your abdomen to swell upwards. Your chest should barely move.
4 As you exhale, let your abdomen flatten.

Give yourself a few minutes to get into a smooth, easy rhythm. As worries and distractions arise, don't hang on to them. Wait calmly for them to float out of your mind – then focus once more on your breathing.

When you feel ready to end the exercise, open your eyes. Allow yourself time to become alert before getting up. With practice, you will begin breathing with your diaphragm quite naturally – and in times of stress, you should be able to correct your breathing without too much effort.

7

Natural remedies

Many people swear by natural remedies such as barley grass juice, noni juice and so on. So do any of them really work? I have been careful to base my assessment of each on scientific facts rather than unproven patient testimonials and biased test results from product manufacturers.

Please remember that what provides relief for one person may actually worsen symptoms for someone else. It is important, therefore, to try out a new remedy for four to six weeks before determining whether or not it is going to be helpful. It's certainly not essential to take remedies, however, especially if you are spending a lot of money on nutritional supplements. Remedies are enormously helpful for some people, but in many cases it is the knowledge that you are doing something to help yourself that provides the most benefit.

Barley grass juice

For many years, people the world over have used barley grass juice as a tonic and natural energy source. However, it wasn't until the start of the twentieth century that it was subjected to scientific research and found to be an excellent source of nutrients required by the body for growth, repair and well-being. Its attributes are largely due to the presence of an important substance called P4D1, which has been shown in laboratory testing to actually repair human DNA – DNA being the carrier of genetic material that occurs in every cell in the body. Damaged DNA leads to ageing, disease and eventual death.

Many experts believe that barley grass has the most balanced nutrient profile of all the green plants. They profess that these nutrients work together as powerful antioxidants to protect our bodies from free radical damage, boost immune system function and improve cardiovascular health.

Dr Howard Lutz, director of the Institute of Preventative

Medicine in Washington, DC, says that barley grass is one of the most incredible products of the age, improving stamina, sexual energy and clarity of thought. He says also that it improves the skin texture and heals the dryness associated with ageing.

Horses and cows, with their long digestive tracts, are able to break down the cellulose fibres of barley grass and so release its nutrients. Unfortunately, our less efficient digestive systems are unable to break down either cellulose or fibre. We cannot, therefore, obtain the nutrients in barley grass simply by eating it, but it can be digested in juice form, and should only be consumed in that way. The harvested grass is washed, 'juiced' and dried at cold temperatures before the resultant powder is hermetically sealed into vacuum-packed bags. Barley grass powders cultured in greenhouse trays or processed in a different way are known to have fewer health benefits.

If you would like to give barley grass juice a try, details of a good supplier are in the Useful addresses section at the back of this book.

Noni juice

Noni juice is derived from the fruit of the *Morinda citrifolia* tree, which commonly flourishes in Polynesia but is most prevalent on the Pacific island of Tahiti. The pungent odour of the fruit when ripening has earned it the informal name of 'vomit fruit'. Its taste is very bitter, too, yet it remains a common food in some Pacific islands. The pulp, bark, leaves and seeds of the noni fruit have been used as a healing tonic for inflammation, constipation, respiratory problems and other ailments for over 2,000 years. More recently in the west, the juice of the fruit has been mixed with more palatable fruit flavours and marketed as 'a miracle in a bottle'. The manufacture of noni juice is consequently a multi-million dollar industry with a loyal following who swear by its health benefits – but there are many inconsistencies in patient testimonials. Experts have also found that the Polynesians themselves only resorted to using the juice as a health tonic when all other avenues had failed.

In 2007, immunologist Dr Jeffrey Galpin reviewed existing noni juice studies (all sponsored by noni juice manufacturers) and made it clear that the manufacturers' claims cannot be backed up. 'It's promoted to do everything with no validation of anything,' he said. There is no doubt that noni fruit powder is rich in carbohydrates, fibre and other beneficial health-giving agents. However, when the juice of the noni fruit was independently analysed in a laboratory, a surprisingly small quantity of these nutrients was detected. Indeed, one medicinal helping was found to contain no more health-giving properties than are present in one orange. Scientists concluded, therefore, that the high nutrient content of noni is stored in the pulp rather than in the juice of the fruit.

France has recently warned prospective customers that there are risks attached to the juice. Some people were found to have severe liver problems after taking the juice, so it should be avoided at all costs if you already have problems with your liver.

The common side effects linked with noni juice are constipation, coughing and wheezing. If you still wish to try taking it, it is recommended that you first get the go-ahead from your doctor. Build up your intake gradually, monitoring the effect very carefully.

Aloe juice

The aloe vera plant has a long history as a folk remedy and is known all over the world as the 'first aid plant' or 'medicine plant'. Both gel and latex can be extracted from the plant, the gel being a clear, jelly-like pulp from the inner part of the leaves and the latex being a bitter yellow substance carried in tiny tubes beneath the outer skin of the leaves. It is the latex that is commonly known as 'aloe juice' and is now widely used to treat a variety of health disorders.

In a range of studies conducted recently, scientists concluded that because aloe juice is packed with a particular combination of nutrients – inclusive of vitamins, minerals and amino acids – it is capable of relieving chronic pain conditions. Also, aloe juice is high in 'basic sugars' (known as mucopolysaccharides), which are normally present in every cell in the body and need replenishment on a regular basis. All these substances, in combination, are thought to make aloe juice an immune system stimulant, a powerful anti-inflammatory and a good analgesic. Aloe juice is also believed to speed up cell repair, which should effectively reduce pain.

Numerous worldwide studies have indicated that aloe juice is capable of improving a wide range of medical conditions. I recently looked at a chronic pain website in which individuals had reported their personal experiences of taking aloe juice, and it's clear that its success varies considerably from person to person. Some individuals report immediate dramatic pain relief, whereas others say that they waited a long time for it to have any effect and in the end there was little or no improvement. I can only assume that it is more successful in those who make positive lifestyle changes, as discussed in this book.

Apart from pink urine, side effects don't normally occur if you follow the label instructions. If you take large quantities of aloe juice over a long period, however, the result can be electrolyte loss, fluid imbalance, intestinal cramps and slow healing of wounds. Further research into aloe juice and its effects would be welcome in the near future. In the meantime, taking the product as instructed can apparently do no harm, and may even be of substantial benefit.

Emu oil

Emu oil, a natural remedy that was used in Australian Aboriginal medicine for hundreds of years, is now famous worldwide as a soothing agent for a variety of health problems. Where chronic pain is concerned, it appears to reduce stiffness and pain. Indeed, scientists claim that in some cases the oil is more effective than NSAIDs such as ibuprofen, and without the side effects.

Emu oil comes in pure oil form or is mixed with other herbs to enhance its efficacy. A topical product, it is massaged into the skin, where it penetrates quickly and completely, healing and nourishing the skin at cellular level. Researchers claim that emu oil, unlike petroleum-based products, has a fatty acid composition similar to the oil in human skin and it is this that enables it to penetrate the skin, giving pain relief in 15 minutes or less. Emu oil also contains vitamins A and E – antioxidants that fight free radical damage (free radicals are unstable molecules that damage our cells, contributing to ageing and age-related diseases). Dr Leigh Hopkins, a clinical professor of pharmacology, even professes that emu oil helps to normalize basic cellular function and allows the body to return to normal healing.

Although I would like to see more scientific evidence regarding the efficacy of emu oil, it is safe to say that it is usually a beneficial treatment for the symptoms of fibromyalgia and other long-term pain disorders.

Cherry juice

Montmorency cherry juice has recently become a popular treatment for a wide range of conditions. The presence of natural antioxidants and powerful substances called anthocyanins (pigments) is what apparently makes it so effective. In fact, it has been found in research to work in the same way as NSAIDs.

Some researchers claim that montmorency cherry juice is as effective at reducing pain as aspirin and ibuprofen, but without the risk of side effects such as stomach irritation, stomach ulcers and kidney damage. It is apparently the antioxidants in these cherries that vastly reduce the risk of side effects. Melatonin – one of its antioxidants – has been subject to much testing on people with sleeping problems, the outcome being that taking melatonin usually causes normal sleep patterns to return. Poor sleep is a major contributing factor in fibromyalgia and this can be improved by taking montmorency cherry juice on a regular basis.

I can verify that drinking montmorency cherry juice is a wonderfully pleasant form of self-medication. Montmorency cherries are available in juice concentrate, and also in capsules, in which the fruit has been freeze-dried into a powder. See the Useful addresses section at the back of this book for details of a good supplier.

Other natural remedies

If you prefer a natural approach to fibromyalgia treatment, it's best to learn as much as you can about any remedy you are considering, and perhaps seek medical advice. For example, if you are already being prescribed a serotonin-enhancing drug, it's vital that you consult your doctor before taking a supplement intended also to boost serotonin. Creating too much serotonin from interactions between drugs can lead to 'serotonin syndrome', a life-threatening disorder which begins with headache, dilated pupils, diarrhoea, restlessness, nausea and fast heartbeat, and can end in confusion, convulsions and death. Numerous drugs and drug combinations have reportedly resulted in this dangerous syndrome.

However, in your research you will find that some studies into the effectiveness of medicinal herbs and nutritional supplements show that they offer significant help, while other studies into the same substances are inconclusive.

The following nutritional supplements are believed to be helpful in treating fibromyalgia.

SAMe (S-adenosylmethionine)

SAMe is an important building block of serotonin. It is found naturally in the body, but it can also be artificially produced in a laboratory from the essential amino acid methionine and adenosine triphosphate (ATP), the latter being the energy-producing chemical found in all the cells in our bodies. The usefulness of SAMe for pain conditions was found accidentally when researchers were looking for a new treatment for depression. Subsequent clinical studies have shown that SAMe can benefit certain conditions often related to fibromyalgia, including the following:

- chronic fatigue syndrome
- anxiety and depression
- bursitis
- tendonitis
- cognitive problems
- chronic lower back pain
- joint problems
- premenstrual syndrome and other problems related to a woman's menstrual cycle.

SAMe is thought to work by crossing the blood–brain barrier (see page 17), where it produces important chemical compounds via a series of reactions. These chemical compounds are the ones involved in pain. Some people are unable to make enough natural SAMe, which means that they feel pain more intensely than others – and this is often the case in fibromyalgia. Replacing the SAMe in the form of a prescription drug or nutritional supplement can, then, benefit many conditions. It is available on prescription in certain countries, and over the counter in others. In the UK, it is not yet available over the counter, but can be purchased online.

If you are using SAMe as a nutritional supplement, it usually comes in 200mg tablets, enteric-coated to protect the stomach. The recommended daily dosage is up to 400mg, but most people prefer 100–200mg, starting with 100mg – half a tablet. Once you have sufficient SAMe in your system you may be able to maintain it with 100mg daily. SAMe supplements are best taken in the morning before or with breakfast. You should feel more alert and energetic within two hours.

5-HTP (5-hydroxytryptophan)
Studies looking into the effectiveness of the supplement 5-HTP – another building block of serotonin – have been inconclusive. Some suggest that 5-HTP boosts endorphin levels in the body

(endorphins work in a similar way to morphine and are known as the body's own natural painkillers), lowering pain intensity, reducing the number of tender points, improving sleep and causing less anxiety and fatigue – all of which are symptoms of serotonin deficiency. Other studies, however, have shown no significant benefit. If you wish to try 5-HTP supplementation, take it for three months; if there is no improvement within that time, stop taking it. There are no side effects linked to this supplement.

Melatonin

This natural hormone is sometimes used to improve sleep patterns, such as after a long-haul flight, to counter jetlag and induce drowsiness. Preliminary research has shown that melatonin may improve the pain and fatigue of fibromyalgia.

There are usually no side effects associated with melatonin. As the main risk is that of daytime sleepiness if taken during daylight hours, you should not drive or operate machinery until you know how the substance affects you.

St John's wort

As this herb can boost the availability of serotonin in the body, it was until recently considered a useful natural treatment for fibromyalgia. Indeed, it was believed to counter depression successfully, promote restful sleep and reduce many other symptoms related to insufficient serotonin. The only drawbacks were thought to be skin reactions in sun-sensitive people and mild stomach discomfort in a few cases, but only if the normal dosage was exceeded. It was therefore believed that St John's wort, when taken with caution, could be of great benefit.

Recent studies have shown, however, that St John's wort can react adversely with certain serotonin-enhancing drugs, creating an overabundance of serotonin. This can potentially result in the life-threatening 'serotonin syndrome' (see page 99).

Drugs that can interact with St John's wort include the following:

- drugs in the Prozac family
- prescription antidepressants
- anti-migraine drugs, in particular sumatriptan (a triptan sulfa medication)
- the painkiller tramadol (brand names Ultram, Zydol and Tramal).

St John's wort also appears to reduce significantly the effectiveness of a wide array of important medications, including cyclosporine and tacrolimus (used in organ transplant), digoxin (used for heart disease), warfarin (for thinning the blood), statins (for reducing high cholesterol), atypical antipsychotics (for schizophrenia), anaesthetics (used in surgical procedures), chemotherapy drugs, oral contraceptives, HIV drugs and tricyclic antidepressants. Some of the interactions provoked by combining St John's wort with other drugs can actually be life-threatening.

Not surprisingly, experts now consider St John's wort unsafe and advise avoiding its use. If you are taking it, it is probably advisable that you stop; ideally your doctor should monitor your drug levels and general condition during the withdrawal process. Remember that it can take a month or more for some drugs to clear from your blood.

DHEA (dehydroepiandrosterone)

The steroid hormone dehydroepiandrosterone (DHEA) has been touted as giving new hope for people with fibromyalgia, chronic fatigue conditions and connective tissue disorders. DHEA occurs naturally in the body and is converted to testosterone, oestrogen and certain other hormones. As we get past the age of 30, however, our natural DHEA levels begin to drop.

Blood tests have shown that people with the disorders mentioned above have DHEA in low supply, probably the result of poor sleep and muscle fatigue. Some studies have indicated that DHEA supplementation may stimulate the immune system and boost levels of IGF-1 (see page 35) and growth hormone. It was therefore concluded that DHEA supplementation could benefit fibromyalgia and similar conditions.

Interestingly, a rigidly controlled double-blind crossover study in 2005 showed that although DHEA supplementation boosts DHEA levels, it does not seem to improve symptoms.[4] In the study, 52 postmenopausal women with fibromyalgia took either 50mg DHEA (the recommended dosage is 25–50mg) or a placebo (simple sugar pill) every day for three months, followed by a one-month break before swapping treatments for a further three months. The results showed that DHEA levels actually tripled in all the volunteers, but not one reported an improvement in her quality of life, pain levels, fatigue, mood, functional impairment or cognitive function. The side effects noted were greasy hair, acne and more body hair – the usual result of an excess of testosterone. The authors of the study believe that long-term DHEA supplementation can increase the risk of breast cancer, too.

DHEA therapy is highly promoted and supplements can be purchased from usual outlets. Until more good-quality research is carried out and the results are clearer, though, DHEA use is not recommended.

Fish oils

In 2009, scientists discovered that our bodies convert the omega 3 essential fatty acids (EFAs) in fish oils into a powerful anti-inflammatory chemical known as resolvin D2. They are now hoping that resolvin D2 will provide the basis for a range of impressive new treatments for inflammatory conditions. Although fibromyalgia is not known as an inflammatory condition, there is a certain amount of inflammation at the nerve endings, which fish oil may help to reduce.

In addition, all oils are a natural source of vitamin E, which is an important antioxidant. Antioxidants are essential to cell life because they mop up destructive 'free radicals' within the body. Unfortunately, when food is processed in some way (that is, when it is prepared or converted by being boiled, for example, and/or having other foodstuffs added), the vitamin E in some unsaturated oils is removed, depriving the body of the vitamin. It is recommended, therefore, that you obtain your fats from natural sources. If you don't think you are getting sufficient essential fatty acids from your diet, supplementation is available in the form of fish oil capsules. Follow the label instructions and take for at least three to six months to see the full effects.

Omega 3 EFAs are obtained from oily fish (such as mackerel, sardines, herring, tuna), vegetable oils, seeds (sunflower, sesame, flax), nuts and avocados. Oils should be stored in a sealed container in a cool, dark place to prevent rancidity.

Evening primrose oil

Although this herbal supplement has long been known as an immune system regulator, recent trials aimed at proving or disproving this claim have been inconclusive. Note that evening primrose oil may be of detriment to people with overactive immune systems, such as in rheumatoid arthritis and lupus, and they are advised to steer clear of it.

If you think it is safe for you to try evening primrose oil, keep in mind that it takes three to six months for the full benefit to be apparent.

Cat's claw

Extracted from a Peruvian vine, cat's claw is widely used in South America for treating joint inflammation and pain. To date there have been no studies in humans, but studies in animals have shown that it can act as an antioxidant and anti-inflammatory. It is available in capsules and teabags; but be careful to select the *uncaria tomentosa* variety, as other types can be toxic. Note that cat's claw can increase the risk of bleeding if taken with blood thinners such as warfarin, heparin or aspirin.

Devil's claw

Devil's claw is derived from an African plant, the roots of which are believed to contain anti-inflammatory and painkilling properties. Although it is widely used for treating rheumatoid arthritis, studies have so far been inconclusive. Like cat's claw, it is available in capsules and teabags, but it should not be used if you have digestive problems and/or a stomach ulcer, as it stimulates stomach acid. If you wish to try devil's claw, ensure that it contains harpagoside, the active ingredient.

Cayenne

Also called capsaicin, cayenne is made from ground chillies and applied externally as a cream to temporarily ease chronic pain conditions. Chillies trigger the release of endorphins – the body's natural painkillers; they also interfere with a chemical responsible for sending pain signals and can actually block pain for a time. Apply cayenne only to unbroken skin and always wash your hands thoroughly after using it.

Ginger

Ginger root shows great potential as it can inhibit the production of the chemicals involved in inflammation and pain. It can be used in generous amounts in cooking and to flavour herbal teas. It also comes in tablet and powder form.

Beware if you are taking blood-thinning drugs such as warfarin and heparin, though, as when combined with ginger they increase the risk of bleeding.

Boswellia

Also known as frankincense, boswellia comes from an Asian gum tree. It has been used in Indian ayurvedic medicine for years to treat the inflammation of arthritis and the muscular pains that come with conditions such as fibromyalgia. However, the results of studies into the efficacy of boswellia have been inconclusive and there is a need for better-quality trials. The side effects linked to boswellia include diarrhoea, a rash or nausea.

Green tea

Green tea contains compounds called phenols, which are believed to work as antioxidants in alleviating pain and reducing inflammation. Note that you shouldn't add milk to your cup of green tea as this could render the phenols useless. As well as the widely available teabags, you can buy green tea in tablet or capsule form.

Peppermint

Prized for its distinctive flavour and medicinal qualities, peppermint is a naturally occurring hybrid of spearmint and water mint. Unlike other mints, however, peppermint contains menthol – a powerful therapeutic ingredient.

Peppermint is often used with success to treat the following conditions:

- *Irritable bowel syndrome* – peppermint oil can be used to great effect for treating the symptoms of IBS, because it can relax the digestive tract. Take one or two enteric-coated peppermint capsules two or three times a day between meals. Each capsule should contain 0.2ml of oil. Many people drink peppermint tea every day as it offers a soothing option to capsules or tinctures.
- *Muscle aches and pains* – peppermint oil, when massaged into the skin, produces a cool, soothing sensation and desensitizes pain messages. Add several drops of undiluted peppermint oil to one tablespoon of neutral carrier oil, such as almond oil, and massage into the affected areas, up to four times a day. To reduce the pain of a headache or migraine, some sources recommend rubbing a mixture of peppermint oil, eucalyptus oil and ethanol (ethyl alcohol) into your forehead and temples.
- *Alleviating tension and fatigue* – the aroma of peppermint oil, when added to bath water, is thought to help you feel less tense and tired. Add a few drops to running water to dissipate the oil.

As well as the oil, peppermint comes as a tincture, soft gel, ointment, dried herbal tea, cream and in capsules. To brew a cup of peppermint tea, use one to two teaspoons of dried peppermint leaves to 8 fluid ounces of water. Pour very hot (not boiling) water over the leaves, cover the cup to prevent the volatile oil from being released, and allow the mixture to steep for ten minutes, before straining.

Rosemary

The leaves and twigs of the rosemary plant can be used for both culinary and medicinal purposes. Herbalists have long used the plant to improve memory, relieve muscle pain and support the circulatory and nervous systems.

Rosemary is available as the dried whole herb, powdered extract (in capsules), tinctures, infusions and a volatile essential oil – the latter for external use only. The total daily intake should not exceed 4–6g of the dried herb. Recommended dosages are as follows:

- *Tea* – three cups daily. Make an infusion by pouring boiling water over the herb and then steeping for three to five minutes. Use 6g of powdered herb to two cups of water. Divide this amount into three small cups and drink over the course of the day.
- *Tincture* (1:5) – 2–4ml taken three times a day.
- *Fluid extract* (1:1 in 45 per cent alcohol) – 1–2ml taken three times a day.

Externally, the essential oil may be used as follows:

- *For massage* – mix two drops of rosemary oil in one tablespoonful of a neutral oil, then massage into a painful area.
- *In the bath* – place ten drops of rosemary oil into warm bathwater for a relaxing bath.

Rosemary is generally considered safe when taken in the recommended doses. However, large quantities of rosemary leaves, because of their volatile oil content, can cause serious side effects, including vomiting, spasms, even coma, and in some cases pulmonary oedema (fluid in the lungs).

Women who are pregnant or breastfeeding should not use rosemary in quantities larger than normally used in cooking. An overdose of rosemary may induce a miscarriage or damage the foetus.

Beta-nicotinamide adenine dinucleotide (NADH)

This natural co-enzyme is present in all the cells in our body, its chief function being the production of energy. In several double-blind randomized trials it was shown to increase dopamine levels, reducing fatigue and improving mental clarity, memory and concentration. Other trials, however, have shown little or no improvement. Better-quality trials are required to demonstrate fully the effects of this supplement. If you wish to try NADH, the recommended dosage is 5–10 mg daily. Coated tablets are said to be the most successful. NADH in supplement form has no significant side effects and there have been no reported drug interactions.

L-theanine

Early studies have indicated that this amino acid, found only in black and green tea, induces alpha brain waves, boosts serotonin levels and increases the secretion of an important chemical called GABA (see pages 22–4). The result is said to be a calming effect and improved relaxation. L-theanine is also believed to lower blood pressure, enhance immune function and improve cognitive performance (concentration, memory and so on). There is actually some evidence that L-theanine protects the brain cells from damage – hence the improved mental clarity – but much further research is required.

This substance is non-toxic and side effect free, even in large doses. You may already be taking it in the form of black tea, but it's best to buy the decaffeinated variety, placing your emphasis on green tea, not black. Drink it in moderation, however, as chemicals are used in the decaffeination process. Green tea is available in capsule form, as well as, of course, the natural tea infusion, using teabags. Pop a slice of lemon into your green tea instead of using milk. Don't drink more than five cups of tea daily, and avoid sweetening with sugar.

Adaptogenic herbs for stress

Approximately two-thirds of all visits to GP surgeries are for stress-related complaints. Stress itself is not an illness, however – it is a fact of life. Going back to when we lived in caves, we were often at risk of attack by wild animals and neighbouring mobs. Stress hormones such as adrenalin, dopamine, norepinephrine and epinephrine were pumped into the body, causing shallower breathing, a faster heart rate, higher blood pressure and sluggish digestion. This prepared the caveman to either stay and fight or turn and take flight – hence the stress response is known as 'fight or flight'. Our bodies still react to threats in the way they did then. In the modern world, the same stress hormones are pumped into our bodies each time something troublesome occurs, and as this happens quite often with some people, they get stuck in a heightened state of readiness.

The events that can trigger that state of readiness, and so chronic stress, include poor sleep, unhealthy diet, chemical toxins and negative life events such as failing at tasks, a poor self-image, an injury, anxiety, and so on. However, herbal experts believe that we can prevent stress hormones from flooding our bodies by taking adaptogenic herbs – plants with properties that enable our bodies to cope better with stress. Adaptogenic herbs actually seem capable of recharging the adrenal glands, the two small organs in the body that most determine stress. Indeed, it is the adrenal glands that pump out stress hormones and so easily become exhausted.

Some of the more important adaptogenic herbs are as follows.

Rhodiola rosea

This adaptogen is claimed to benefit the adrenal glands and also believed to boost levels of serotonin, norepinephrine and dopamine, and is therefore thought to greatly benefit fibromyalgia. Rhodiola rosea is often used to treat depression, headaches, migraines, muscle spasm, fatigue and seasonal affective disorder (known as SAD, in which a lack of sunlight causes low mood). Cognitive function, such as memory, clear thinking and concentration, is also said to be improved by this herb.

Ashwaganda

Often called Indian ginseng, this adaptogenic herb is viewed as a tonic, nerve calmer and sedative. It seems to help rebalance the immune system, and can reduce anxiety and other psychological disorders.

Asian ginseng

Also considered a tonic, Asian ginseng is said to be a great strengthener for people with weakness of the muscles, voice and constitution. It is also thought to improve a person's ability to cope with stress, to improve practical function and enhance mental alertness.

American ginseng

This is considered a tonic for a hotter, more aggressive personality. It has many of the same constituents as Asian ginseng and its effect on the body is similar.

Siberian ginseng

This adaptogen is not actually a ginseng, but has similar properties. It has been shown in studies to normalize the response to physical and mental stress. People who take it report greater mental awareness, enhanced physical performance and improved work quality.

Licorice root

Licorice root is said to improve immune system function and evince a stimulating effect on the adrenal glands, which tend to be exhausted where there is stress and pain. This adaptogen can, however, contribute to high blood pressure in some people. If you decide to try it, it's best to have your blood pressure checked on a regular basis.

Useful addresses

General
Fibromyalgia Association UK
Head Office
Training and Enterprise Centre
Applewood Grove
Cradley Heath B64 6EW
Tel.: 0844 826 9022 (office);
    0844 887 2444 (helpline, 10 a.m. to 4 p.m., Monday to Friday)
Email: charity@fmauk.org
Website: www.fmauk.org
Fibromyalgia Association UK is a registered charity administered by unpaid volunteers. It was established to provide information and support to sufferers and their families; a free information pack is available on request. There is also a link on the website to a forum where you can receive support and advice from others with fibromyalgia. In addition, the Association provides medical information for professionals.

Mrs Janet Horton (Fibromyalgia Association UK Trustee)
Helpline: 0844 887 2450 (10 a.m. to 12 noon, Monday and Friday)
For fibromyalgia-related benefit advice.

Fibromyalgia Support Northern Ireland
The Vine Centre
193 Crumlin Road
Belfast BT14 7DX
Tel.: 0844 8269024 (helpline, 10.30 a.m. to 4 p.m., Monday to Friday)
Text: 07549 838800 (for urgent enquiries when out and about; no abbreviations please)
Website: www.fmsni.org.uk
This organization is dedicated to raising fibromyalgia awareness and supporting people with fibromyalgia.

UK Fibromyalgia
(associated with the Fibromyalgia Association UK)
7 Ashbourne Road
Bournemouth BH5 2JS
Website: www.ukfibromyalgia.com
Visit the forum: http://www.ukfibromyalgia.com/forums
Facebook Page: www.facebook.com/fibromyalgia.uk
Twitter: www.twitter.com Search @ukfibromyalgia
Awareness Raising Group: www.facebook.com/groups/UKFibromyalgia/
Private Discussion Group: www.facebook.com/groups/UKFibromyalgia Private/

For fibromyalgia information and advice, experts' comments and more. Providers of the monthly fibromyalgia-related *FaMily* magazine.

FibroAction
46 The Nightingales
Newbury
Berkshire RG14 7UJ
Tel.: 0844 443 5422
Website: www.fibroaction.org
This charitable organization aims to provide information about fibromyalgia. There is also a FibroAction online community where you can get more news, including information about events and ongoing research.

Fibromyalgia Shop
Website: www.fibromyalgiashop.co.uk
This is a new online shop aimed at sufferers of fibromyalgia. Its mission is to provide a one-stop location to source all fibromyalgia requirements, to raise awareness and at the same time raise funds for UK Fibromyalgia support groups. They have, for example, over 50 fibromyalgia-specific books with the very best discounts.

National Fibromyalgia Association
2121 S. Towne Centre
Suite 300
Anaheim
California CA 92806
Tel.: 714 921 0150
Website: www.fmaware.org
This members-only website gives information on support groups and FM community events from Canada to California. There is also the monthly *Fibromyalgia AWARE* magazine.

Pain Log
Website: www.painsupport.co.uk/enewsletter/painlevelslog.pdf
This site provides a 'pain log' to help you keep track of your pain and find out what affects it. The log can then be used in medical consultations to show your doctor how your pain affects you.

Legal

Andrew Isaacs Solicitors Ltd
7 Shaw Wood Business Park
Shaw Wood Way
Leger Way
Doncaster DN2 5TB
Tel.: 01302 349 480
Fax: 01302 368 572
Website: www.andrewisaacs.co.uk
For information and advice regarding possible litigation claims.

Brian Barr Solicitors
Grosvenor House
Agecroft Road
Manchester M27 8UW
Tel.: 0161 737 9248
Fax: 0161 637 4946
Website: www.brianbarr.co.uk
The solicitor Brian Barr is familiar with fibromyalgia and has represented sufferers in making successful claims.

Natural remedies

CherryActive Ltd
Unit 18, Mill Farm Business Park
Millfield Road
Hanworth
Middlesex TW4 5PY
Tel.: 08451 705705 (9 a.m. to 5 p.m., Monday to Friday; also for ordering in the UK)
Website: www.cherryactive.co.uk
International orders: +44 20 8744 5291
Order CherryActive juice and capsules via telephone or the website.

Nutri Centre
Unit 3, Kendal Court
Kendal Avenue
London W3 0RU
Tel.: 020 8752 8450 (for general and mail-order enquiries)
Website: www.nutricentre.com
There is a new website specifically for ordering, <www.nutribeautyproducts.com>. Login details will be necessary. Phone the general number for further details or search the website. A wide range of good-quality vitamins, minerals and supplements are provided through this organization, as well as beauty products and related items.

Green Ways International
Tel: (mobile) 00 34 686 739 300 (ask for Madhu)
Email: mdhankani25@yahoo.com
For good quality barley grass juice products at reasonable prices.

Vitamins Direct Ltd
PO Box 621
York House
Wetherby Road
York YO26 0EX
Tel.: 0800 634 9985 (freephone, 8 a.m. to 8 p.m., Monday to Friday; 9 a.m. to 6 p.m., Saturday and Sunday)
Website: www.vitaminsdirectonline.co.uk
Vitamins Direct is a leading supplier of good-quality vitamins, minerals and supplements.

Other organizations

Arthritis Research UK
Copeman House
St Mary's Gate
Chesterfield
Derbyshire S41 7TD
Tel.: 0300 790 0400
Website: www.arthritisresearchuk.org

Backcare – the Charity for Healthier Backs
16 Elmtree Road
Teddington
Middlesex TW11 8ST
Tel.: 020 8977 5474 (national office, 9 a.m. to 4.30 p.m., Monday to Thursday); 0845 130 2704 (helpline)
Website: www.backcare.org.uk

Carers UK
20 Great Dover Street
London SE1 4LX
Tel.: 020 7378 4999 (office); 0808 808 7777 (adviceline, 10 a.m. to noon/2 p.m. to 4 p.m., Wednesday and Thursday)
Website: www.carersuk.org
Carers UK is the voice of carers. The association gives support to those who provide unpaid care by looking after an ill, frail or disabled family member, friend or partner.

Let's Talk Pain
Website: www.letstalkpain.com
This is a coalition of leading chronic pain advocacy groups in America, focused on increasing awareness and improving understanding of pain management. It brings together organizations representing those affected by pain: patients, caregivers and healthcare professionals.

Pain Support
www.painsupport.co.uk
This site provides access to a monthly email newsletter and pain-relief 'Tool Kit'; two collections of tips on relaxation may be downloaded free; and there are links to a Discussion Forum and Contact Club, as well as to Facebook.

References

1 Daniel J. Clauw, Richard H. Gracely, Seong-Ho Kim, 'Dynamic levels of glutamate within the insula are associated with improvements in multiple pain domains in fibromyalgia', *Arthritis and Rheumatism*, 2008, 58(3).

2 M. E. Powers, S. E. Borst, S. C. McCoy, R. Conway and J. Yarrow, 'The effects of gamma aminobutyric acid on growth hormone secretion at rest and following exercise', *Medicine and Science in Sports and Exercise*, 2003, 35(5), Supplement, p. S271.

3 F. A. Beebe, R. L. Barkin and S. Barkin, 'A clinical and pharmacologic review of skeletal muscle relaxants for musculoskeletal conditions', *American Journal of Therapy*, 2005, 12(2), pp. 151–71.

4 A. Finckh et al., 'A randomized controlled trial of dehydroepiandrosterone in postmenopausal women with fibromyalgia', *Journal of Rheumatology*, 2005, 32(7), pp. 1336–40.

Further reading

Stacie L. Bigelow, *Fibromyalgia: Simple Relief Through Movement*, New York: John Wiley, 2000.

Christine Craggs-Hinton, *Living with Fibromyalgia*, new edition, London: Sheldon Press, 2010.

Christine Craggs-Hinton, *The Fibromyalgia Healing Diet*, new edition, London: Sheldon Press, 2008.

Clair Davies, Amber Davies and David G. Simons, *The Trigger Point Therapy Workbook: Your Self-Treatment Guide for Pain Relief*, second edition, Oaklands, CA: New Harbinger Publications, 2004.

Chris Jenner, *Fibromyalgia and Myofascial Pain Syndrome: A Practical Guide to Getting on With Your Life*, Oxford: How To Books, 2011.

Ginevra Liptan, *Figuring out Fibromyalgia: Current Science and the Most Effective Treatments*, Kindle edition, Portland, OR: Visceral Books, 2011.

Dawn A. Marcus and Atul Deodhar, *The Woman's Fibromyalgia Toolkit: Manage Your Symptoms and Take Control of Your Life*, New York: Diamedica, 2012.

Roland Staud and Christine Adamec, *Fibromyalgia for Dummies*, New York: John Wiley, 2007.

Index